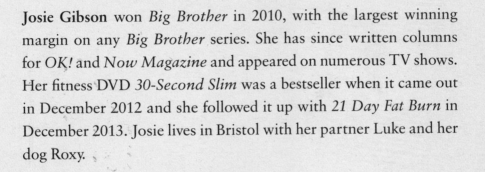

**Josie Gibson** won *Big Brother* in 2010, with the largest winning margin on any *Big Brother* series. She has since written columns for *OK!* and *Now Magazine* and appeared on numerous TV shows. Her fitness DVD *30-Second Slim* was a bestseller when it came out in December 2012 and she followed it up with *21 Day Fat Burn* in December 2013. Josie lives in Bristol with her partner Luke and her dog Roxy.

# The
# JOSIE
# GIBSON
## diet

Love Food, Get Slim, Stay Slim

MACMILLAN

First published 2014 by Macmillan
an imprint of Pan Macmillan, a division of Macmillan Publishers Limited
Pan Macmillan, 20 New Wharf Road, London N1 9RR
Basingstoke and Oxford
Associated companies throughout the world
www.panmacmillan.com

ISBN 978-1-4472-6061-5

This book is intended as a reference volume only, not as a medical
manual. The information given here is designed to help you make informed
decisions about your health. It is not intended as a substitute for any treatment
that you may have been prescribed by your doctor. If you suspect you have a
medical problem, we urge you to seek competent medical help.

Mention of specific companies, organizations or authorities in this book does not
imply endorsement of the publisher, nor does mention of specific companies, organizations
or authorities in the book imply that they endorse the book. Addresses, websites and
telephone numbers given in this book were correct at the time of going to press.

1 3 5 7 9 8 6 4 2

A CIP catalogue record for this book is available from the British Library.

Printed and bound by CPI Group (UK) Ltd, Croydon, CR0 4YY

Visit **www.panmacmillan.com** to read more about all our books
and to buy them. You will also find features, author interviews and
news of any author events, and you can sign up for e-newsletters
so that you're always first to hear about our new releases.

This book is dedicated to:

My dear friend and ghostwriter Clare O'Reilly. She has stuck by me and my over-excited mind and made sense of everything I said. I can't thank you enough (even for giving up on the sugar). You are a legend, Thelma, and have made me see that anything is possible . . . Love Louise.

My friends and family, thank you for always being there, and Kate for the gorgeous recipes.

Everyone who is on or about to start a weight loss journey they will never forget.

Love Josie xx

# Contents

Letter from Josie                                           1

Step 1 Get Your Brain On Board                              3

Introduction                                                5
1. Work Out Why You're Here                                11
2. What Kind of Eater Are You?                             21
3. Figure Out Your X-Factors – Stress, Genes and
   Your Body Type                                          31
4. Find Your Motivation                                    45
5. Believe You're Worth It                                 57

Step 2 How to Eat Lots of Healthy Food *and* Lose Weight  65

Introduction                                               67
6. Why the Diet Works                                      75
7. Starting the Diet – What to Eat and Meal Plans          99
8. The Recipes                                            125
9. How to Stay Motivated – Beating the Cravings and
   Sugar Withdrawal                                        191

**Step 3  How to Burn Fat and Shape Up** 215

Introduction 217
10. Getting Started 219
11. High-Intensity Exercise 225

**Step 4  A Lifetime Plan** 231

12. Keeping Your Nerve and Coping with Plateaus 233
13. Enjoy the Journey and Celebrate Success 243

Final letter from Josie 253

# Letter from Josie

My dear muckers,

What you're holding in your hands is your wake-up call. Well, technically it's a book – but indulge me for a sec, all right? I'm Josie Gibson, the fat bird who won *Big Brother* back in the day, then lost over five stone in six months – that's five dress sizes. And before we go any further: no, I didn't get a gastric bypass; I got off my big arse, moved more, ate less and educated myself on what I was stuffing into my body.

If someone had told me a year ago I'd be writing a book about how I did it – and how you can do it too – I'd have choked on my carrot stick. But here it is. If you really want it to, this book can change your life. It will tell you every detail of my journey: what I ate and drank; my workout regime; how I shopped; what I learned; how my body coped physically and my mind coped emotionally; and, most importantly – the holy grail of weight-loss – how I've managed to keep the weight off for good and not pile it all back on again. In these pages I've shared every coping mechanism I developed, every tip and trick I figured out to keep going. I'll teach you everything you need to know about grub, from what you should be putting in your cakehole to how the big food producers make their profits from your shopping habits.

But there are a few rules to explain before I start sharing my secrets. Firstly, don't even read any further unless you really – and I mean *really* – want to change your body and your life for good. I'm the 5ft 11in, size 10, blonde proof that it is possible to drop five dress sizes from a 20 to a 10 and get the body you've always longed for. Getting off your backside and losing weight isn't easy, but it can be done. And as me old fruit Kelly Clarkson reminded us: what doesn't kill you makes you stronger – both physically and mentally.

Secondly, there's no quick fix to anything in life, whether it's getting your broadband connected, healing a broken heart or losing weight. I've changed many things in my life, from my hair colour to my bra size to my men. But the biggest and hardest thing I've ever had to change is my relationship with food. I spent far too many years of my life not even realizing I found comfort at the bottom of a bag of chips, a tub of Ben & Jerry's and bottles of rosé wine. But finally understanding this didn't mean I was able to change overnight. No matter what anyone promises, pretty much everything that's worthwhile takes time, effort, hard work, love, a good old-fashioned dose of determination and a bit of help from your Aunty Josie.

Thirdly, if I can turn things around, anyone can. It's never too late, you're never too old and never too fat, OK?

Your Aunty Josie xxx

# STEP 1

# Get Your Brain On Board

# Introduction

If you want to change your waistline for good, you need to change what's in your head too, and that's as big a task as ditching cakes and biscuits. Just changing what you put in your gob and how much you move around might help you lose weight in the short term, but unless you tackle how you feel about food and the role it plays in your life, heart and mind in the long term, you'll always revert to type and end up putting the weight back on.

Until you are really honest with yourself about your relationship with food, the minute you stop whatever diet you're on, you'll regain the weight you've lost and then some. This is the reason diets don't really work. That's why we're not diving straight into the diet section and why I want you to read the chapters in Step 1 first.

Being big is as much a mindset as it is a number on the scales. It becomes second nature to say no to anything too physical, to constantly try to hide your stomach by folding your arms across it. To dread getting naked in front of anyone. To hate the hot days when everyone else is in shorts or little dresses and you're in your baggy trousers so you can hide your cellulite. After all, why draw even more attention to yourself than you do already? Why spend hours shopping for clothes when nothing fits? Why even bother trying to chat up the fit bloke in the bar?

I felt that being fat was an invisibility cloak and one that grew to feel as familiar as a comfy pair of slippers. You can be the funniest girl in the room and the Johnny Depp lookalike will spend his whole night laughing with you, touching your arm and holding your gaze. But just when you start to think he might not mind that your thigh is as thick as his waist, the lights will come up, he'll hug you and leave – taking home the size 8 hottie in the corner, some of your funniest jokes and that little bit of self-esteem you were just starting to enjoy. For me, being fat meant I was always the best mate, never the lover. The problem is, though, once you've grown to accept that, you start to make less of an effort and it becomes a self-fulfilling prophecy. A bit like the depression and obesity cycle, of which more later. What's the point of wearing those painfully high heels on a night out? No bloke's going to look at you, so you might as well go for your comfy flats. Why spend ages doing your hair when the blokes in the club are always going to see you as a mate rather than a potential girlfriend? You might as well just scrape it back and get down the pub in time for happy hour.

I've always had fat mates and thin mates, and while they've always just looked at me as Josie, I only ever shared my deepest, darkest fears and secrets with my fellow larger-than-life best friend J. We met when we were teenagers and used to work the summer seasons in Ayia Napa together. We'd go out on the lash calling ourselves 'The Big Girls', joking with blokes that there was too much of us for them to handle. But in secret, in those searingly honest moments you only have with your closest friends who you know will never judge you after a few bevvies, we'd talk about how we longed to be loved and how we'd love to be part of a couple like the ones we saw on our nights out. You know the ones I mean:

he's tall and handsome, she's petite and sexy, they walk down the street holding hands, or maybe he has his hand placed delicately in the small of her back. They both know they're good-looking; he's proud to have her on his arm and she's proud to be there.

J and I both had boyfriends who treated us badly and we honestly put it down to our weight. From my first bloke Kevin to John James on *Big Brother*, all I ever wanted was someone who'd be proud of being my man. Someone who thought I was worth showing off because they loved me. And I never felt that way with either of them if I'm totally honest, but the problem was probably with me. When I was overweight, I could barely stand to see myself naked, never mind anyone else copping an eyeful. The thought of sex when you're a size 18 or 20 is about as nerve wracking as it gets. I remember losing my virginity at sixteen and a size 16 and being more terrified about being seen naked than I did about the thought I was about to do it for the first time. It was all I could stand to look at myself naked after a bath, asking someone else to look at me in the buff and pretend they enjoyed it seemed above and beyond the call of duty. And that feeling didn't change with age. The older I got the more grateful I felt whenever any bloke agreed to have sex with me – not that they were forming a queue round the block. And entering the boudoir on anything less than an even playing field can leave one of you feeling crap and undermined, often while the other carries on in blissful ignorance.

When I got my first long-term boyfriend in my late teens, I was so delighted he wanted to sleep in the same bed as me, let alone touch me, I worked my backside off in bed making sure he had the time of his life – not giving a second thought to the fact it's a team sport and by the end of it we should both have had a good time. Pretty, thin girls can just lie there because their blokes feel like they've won the lottery getting to bed them, whereas I used to have an overwhelming sense my bloke was going to come to his senses as soon as he saw me in the buff. That he'll have his clothes back on and be bolting for the door before I could get my socks back on. I had to work twice as hard in the boudoir to make up for the fact I wasn't much to look at naked.

As if I didn't have a low enough opinion of myself, seeing my first boyfriend's eyes linger on my belly and thighs and bum whenever we made love left me diving for the light switch – pretending I was freezing to get under the covers and hide the bits I hated as fast as I could.

That's the bottom line really (pardon the pun). My self-esteem was at such rock bottom when I was bigger that having sex just made it worse.

Whether any of my boyfriends really felt ashamed of me and my size or whether I pushed my insecurities and body image problems onto them I'll never know, but looking back I'm pretty sure I loathed myself more than they ever did. I just hid how I felt and pretended it didn't bother me – that I liked being big.

You see, that's the biggest lie us fatties tell ourselves right there. I'm guilty of it myself. I'd pretend I liked having an inch or three to pinch, that I was happy being the big girl because I had a big personality to match. That having a big ol' booty meant I had more to shake. But it's all total arse – literally and metaphorically. No one likes being fat. No one. Fact. It's unhealthy, restrictive, physically tiring and means you miss out on living life to the full.

The hardest part of making the life change I have been through is changing what was in my head, rather than what was on my shopping list. I'd thought about losing weight before and had managed to lose a bit here and there through dieting or as a result of a broken heart, but I could never sustain it because my head wasn't in the right place. I didn't like myself and so I didn't think I was worth the effort it was going to take to shift the weight.

The fact is, you're the most important thing you own in this entire world. But the reality is that you've probably been treating your pet, your car or that busybody you hate in accounts better than you've been treating yourself, whether it's by gorging on junk food and chocolate or smoking and drinking. Whether it's through lousy portion control or lack of exercise, if you're overweight, you're slowly killing yourself. Taking better care of everyone and everything else rather than yourself will only hasten you into a hospital ward with weight-related illnesses like diabetes, liver problems or a heart condition. You owe it to your family, your mates, hell, even your pet to be in the best nick you can be. Most of all you owe it to yourself, and I want you to remember that.

# ONE

# Work Out Why You're Here

If you're overweight, chances are you've tried diets before and none of them have worked long term. I want this time to be different. So before I start telling you how to lose weight, before you can lose the extra pounds you're lugging around, you need to understand how you got here in the first place. Knowing why you have the relationship you do with food will help you break the bad habits of a lifetime. So take a deep breath: we're going to work out why you piled on the pounds in the first place.

I was always one of those big birds who hid behind the idea that I had a slow metabolism. Or I'd tell people I was big-boned. While there may have been some truth in both those excuses, the reality is that I was a chubber because I ate and drank far too much, far too often and most of it was crap. Not to mention the fact that when you're overweight it hurts your joints to exercise.

I might have started life as your average 7lb 1oz baby, but my dear dad Danny gave me the sweetest tooth in Yate (19 miles outside Bristol if you ever fancy a visit) by weaning me on rice pudding. Even now I'd sell my soul for a bowl of Ambrosia's finest with a dollop of strawberry jam on top. As soon as I started school and went onto free school meals, things got worse. I've always been greedy and never felt full very quickly. Now I realized that if I got my head down and ate fast, I could be on seconds of cottage pie, fish and chips, spaghetti bolognese or chocolate sponge and custard while everyone else was still on firsts.

You see, my mum Mandy was never a morning person, and I was used to getting my own breakfast from about the age of five, whether it was a few custard creams, four slices of white toast with butter and strawberry jam or a dry bowl of Frosties. Having eaten my sugar-filled breakfast early, in front of kids' TV, I was always starving by the time the lunch bell went at school.

Growing up, meal times at home were sporadic at best. After school I'd play out in the streets or on the green in front of our house with my mates, and then they'd all be called in for their tea, leaving me on my own. Eventually I'd amble home to make myself a banana and sugar sandwich when it started getting dark or I started getting hungry, whichever came first. My parents weren't neglectful intentionally; they just had a lot going on and I was fiercely independent and wanted to do everything myself.

There were never specially prepared dinners around the table with conversations about school, homework or what we'd be doing at half-term or in the summer holidays. Every meal time, be it breakfast, lunch or dinner, was always on the hoof, always an afterthought rather than a priority. Some families can set their watches by their meal times; if we'd tried that, it would have made us days late for everything.

We did a big shop when we could. Mum would load me and my little brother Harry into a double trolley and I'd sit there making him giggle till he spat his dummy out while we made our way round the aisles, but all the best bits would always be eaten in a day or so, leaving the Primula cream cheese, tinned corn beef and all the stuff that had been on special offer or near its sell-by date, which Mum had grabbed as a bargain. She didn't have much money so Mum would always buy things that were cheap and would last a long time.

We certainly weren't the ones doing a weekly shop with a list of meals planned for every day of the week. No, we were the ones hiding from the security guard, eating as much as we could on the way round while Mum stuffed all the expensive things like smoked cheese and garlic sausage in our coat pockets or Jaffa Cakes down Harry's little pants.

When I started school, I'd come home not knowing whether there'd be enough money for a takeaway, usually from the chipper or a Chinese, or whether I'd be making my own tea out of whatever I could find and reach in the cupboards, fridge and freezer – usually three or four rounds of salad-cream sandwiches on white Sunblest with a couple of packets of crisps and some Bourbon biscuits for pudding.

So scranning down as much food as I could at school dinners made sense for us all. I didn't go hungry and Mum – who'd never been taught how to cook – didn't have to hear me whinging about not having enough food. It might not have been everyone's cup of tea. But when I heard tales of friends who weren't allowed out because they hadn't finished their tea or got a slap for coming in late to a cold dinner that had been sitting there for hours, it made me appreciate what I had. Not only nice home-cooked grub for lunch at school, which had been made with care, attention and compassion, but also free rein to come in and out when I wanted after school and free access to the cupboards, fridge and freezer. It meant I could stay out as long as I liked and eat what I wanted, when I wanted. If I fancied eating a whole pack of garlic sausage, sat on the sofa watching Phillip Schofield and Andi Peters, no one stopped me. *Grange Hill* and some Golden Wonder? Don't mind if I do.

I'd split my weekends and my meal times between our council house and my mum's parents' place, Grove House, a few miles away. Nan and my pops had acres of land and a few horses out the back. Grove House was like our family's Grand Central Station: there was always someone coming or going at any time of day or night. It would have made more sense for Nan to install a revolving door rather than a front one, which incidentally was always on the latch. Mum would drop me over if she had things to do and I'd be met with the warm smell of Nan's stew and Pops' stale tobacco smoke whatever time of day I let myself in.

Nan was the stew queen in my eyes. She called them stews because she was old school, born in 1938; she didn't believe in sugar-coating stuff. If Jamie Oliver were to serve her stew he'd probably call it country-style chicken or melt in your mouth succulent shin braise. But Nan was no Jamie, so it was always just 'stew'. No one ever dared ask what kind or what was in it. The catch-all title meant it didn't matter if the ingredients changed. No meat or vegetable in the name meant she could mix it up however she wanted, and we'd accept it as being the same dish whatever was in it. There'd always be a huge pot of it simmering away on the Aga come rain or shine. Most people offer visitors coffee or tea; Nan and Pops offered them stew.

An old guy, Douglas, used to live in one of the outhouses on their land out the back. He'd been there ever since I remembered, but it was only when I was grown up that I learned he'd been a homeless tramp. He'd knocked on the door at some point in the 1970s asking for a cup of coffee or tea on a cold winter's day. Nan gave him a bowl of stew and he stayed for the remaining fifteen years of his life. Now if that's not stew with superpowers, I don't know what is.

Nan's stew was tender, tasty and made all the better with a chunk of fresh French bread spread with Stork. Coming from a home where dinner was an afterthought, no meal was ever planned and the closest we got to slow cooking was walking rather than running back from the takeaway, it was comforting.

Nan knew Harry and I needed feeding, and she didn't remember at the last minute like Mum sometimes did. She knew when she went to bed the previous night what she was going to make us for tea – stew, obviously. I never felt like an inconvenience when Nan cooked for us. Eating a steaming hot bowl of her stew while she sat beside us smoking a fag or mopped the floor around our chairs telling us to eat up before it got cold, we felt remembered, important and cherished. Harry, despite only ever eating cereal when he was tiny at home, would always tuck heartily into a bowl of her stew, something that annoyed Mum and pleased Nan in equal measure.

As I got older and spent more time at Grove House, Nan and I would go on day trips – which were always food related. Whether it be bombing up the M4 in her clapped-out old white Land Rover, trying the full English in every service station on the way, or heading down to Devon and sampling cream teas for the length of the M5, every day trip with Nan involved eating as much as possible, as quickly as possible.

We were poor growing up, but Nan, my formative food mentor, always made sure we were fed good British food. Growing up as one of thirteen, whose parents had survived the First World War, she and her family really didn't have a pot to piss in, let alone extra cash to spend on organic meat and veg, and that right there is the kicker. Levels of obesity in the UK increase in line with deprivation. In short, if you left school with few qualifications and have a menial unskilled job, your risk of obesity (if you're not there yet) is much higher than that of the lawyer or teacher who lives down the road.

People on lower incomes, working-class folk, are far more likely to end up obese than the upper-class lot round the corner. If you live in a deprived area, you're more likely to be obese, and with Yate ranked a glamorous forty-fifth on a list of the fifty worst towns in the UK to live in, and a mum and nan who both left school without a single qualification to their name, you could say I was the underdog from the minute I took my first breath.

Nan and I would drive as far as Glastonbury (thirty-five miles away) to go to her favourite fish and chip shop, Whitstone's on Kilver Street, opposite the Blackthorn Cider factory. We'd drive hundreds if not thousands of miles every year on our Fish and Chip Challenge, as we called it, trying to find the best battered cod within a 200-mile radius – peeling off crisp batter and flaking white cod, pouring on vinegar and seeing how long it took before the chips started getting soggy. Nan and her mates would always debate who served the best fish and chips all the way along the M5 corridor; she'd always claim she knew best because she had me there to back her up and nod in sage agreement.

But it wasn't just Nan who spoiled me rotten and helped me expand my young waistline; my dear old pops was no better. He kept a money tin on top of the telly which he called Josie's sweetie fund. He asked everyone who came round to donate a few coins, so I blame him for funding my addiction to Irn-Bru bars during my formative years. I wasn't much more than eight when my Pops passed away. Nan went a bit funny in the head after losing the love of her life. Her daughter, my aunty Ria, died after battling leukemia a few years later and it was all too much for her. She ended up being arrested as a drug courier, though she always said she was duped and I believe her. She went on the run for more than a decade and is now serving out her sentence in her late seventies.

So with Dad weaning me on rice pudding, Mum never learning to cook, Nan being a connoisseur of deep-fried or full-fat anything and my pops' sweetie fund, the writing was on the wall. I was destined to end up at nine stone when I was just nine years old.

It didn't help that we never did any physical activity as a family. The most exercise I got was every Saturday morning when I'd sit on my sleeping bag at the top of the stairs with Harry sitting behind me, struggling to get his little arms round my ever-expanding podgy waist, then we'd use it as a mat to slide down the stairs like we were on a helter-skelter. Mum would get some of her weekly exercise getting in and out of bed to tell us to keep it down.

Mum was always trim herself, as actually when I was at school she'd spend hours breaking in horses for Nan and Pops – gruelling physical work. Our whole family would go to horse shows and we'd watch Mum and my aunties compete. They tried to make me into a good rider and I spent hours in Nan's paddock falling off, getting back on and giving it a go, determined not to let the side down. I'd have given anything to be as good a rider as my cousins. But I was too big for my age and too heavy for the horses we had. At the horse shows, I'd inevitably find myself hanging out by the ice-cream and burger vans, making myself feel better with food while the rest of my family competed.

One summer, Mum was determined to make me a rider and even got me some private lessons, which was a real stretch for a mum on benefits. She'd tried for years to teach me, but my family's idea of a lesson was to put me on a wild horse and whack its arse, and she finally realized that we might need some outside help from a professional. When we got to the riding school, I couldn't even get on the horse. Mum, the instructor and my aunty gathered round to try to help me up. I grabbed the saddle hard, trying to pull myself onto my pony with all my might, but I was so tense I broke wind really loudly in all their faces. I'd been sick with nerves all morning and with the rest of the kids teasing me for the remaining forty-five minutes of the lesson, it proved in my nine-year-old mind that I was far better off watching the horse shows rather than competing in them. I never got back on a horse and from then on restricted my exercise to the stairs and the sleeping bag.

When Harry's squeals of laughter would get too loud on a Saturday morning, Mum would stir from her pit and threaten to wallop me if I didn't keep it down. I'd abandon my weekend activity in favour of a packet of Real McCoy's in front of *SM:tv Live* or *Scooby Doo*.

When I used to see mums, dads and kids out on bike rides together, I'd think they were all weird do-gooders. I'd look at them on their bikes and think: 'There you all go, pretending to be all holier than thou – what secrets are you lot really hiding?' I'd look at the dad up front and be sure he was too good to be true. The idea of doing something physical as a family was such an alien concept to me that I was sure any family I saw keeping fit was using it as a cover-up, a ruse for something untoward.

When you're big, people look at you like it's all your own fault, and in my case it was. No one forced that third Chelsea bun down my neck on the way back from school. No one made me sit and watch *Blue Peter* with three sherbet Dip Dabs instead of going for long walks in the field by our council house. But by the time I realized I was big because I ate too much, probably when I was around eight years old, I didn't know how to undo it. I loved my tangerines as much as my scones and cream, but no one told me one of those things was good for me and the other wasn't. I craved sweets and loved cake, but no one told me my sweet tooth came from being weaned on rice pudding instead of stewed carrots. Mum, the headmistress and school nurse did get together to try to sort me out

– and part of their plan was that I'd have a healthy lunch. Trouble was that Mum would give me a packed lunch consisting of things like chopped carrot, tomato and cucumber, which I found so boring it would take me the whole lunch break to choke it down, meaning I'd missed out on playing with my friends. As a result, healthy food felt like a punishment.

I knew athletes weren't fat, but I presumed they were born their way and I'd pulled the short straw and been born my way. Mum couldn't afford to buy me a bike, I'd outgrown the set of wheels handed down by my mate across the road and I was too big and embarrassed to join any of the sports clubs at school. At senior school I'd fake asthma attacks and pretend I was on my period so I didn't have to take part in games. Or I'd spend hours the night before in my bed drawing really lifelike bruises on my legs and arms as an excuse not to join in hockey. I'm not in the blame game and I try to focus more on the future than the past; but if you look back, if you ask your family, I guarantee you'll be able to find the trigger that set you off on the path that got you to the size you are now.

# Homework

To help you work out what role food played in your life when you were growing up, ask yourself the following questions:
- Did you care or even think about what you were putting in your mouth?
- Was food plentiful and could you help yourself to anything?
- Did you not know where your next meal was coming from and so overate at any opportunity to compensate?

- Was food used in celebration or as an emotional crutch for bad news, or both?
- Who was in charge of portion control?
- Could you always have seconds?
- Did you always get pudding whether you ate your tea or not?
- Did you do lots of clubs at school and go out on your bike for hours?
- Did you get the bus everywhere, or go for long walks for a gossip with your mates?

This isn't supposed to be *Mastermind*, but I guarantee if you take your time, answer all these questions honestly and look long and hard at your family circumstances, relationships and life journey up to this point, you'll start to understand how and why you got to this place and how your relationships with food were formed. And once you understand that, you can start to figure out how to undo the negative patterns associated with food that have got you to where you are now.

# TWO

# What Kind of Eater Are You?

As well as understanding where your issues with grub come from, finding out what kind of eater you are will help you break bad old habits and form healthy new ones. I was an emotional eater. Good news, bad news, fights, rows, celebrations, breakdowns – I can relate any point on the emotional roller coaster to a time when I was stuffing food in my face. Like the time I celebrated with three burgers on the jog when I was a teenager after getting the whole audience singing while we were waiting for Oasis to come on at Glastonbury. Or the time I ate two kebabs to console myself after realizing I'd lost my passport hours before a holiday to Turkey with the girls. The quiz below will help you identify what kind of eater you are, which is the first step in retraining your mind to get your emotional relationship with food onto an even, healthier keel. You'll learn to separate your emotions from food rather than always keeping them linked.

**1. You've had a crappy day at work, laddering your tights on the bus and breaking your heel on your lunch break. Do you:**

a) stop for some Ben & Jerry's and a bottle of white wine on the way home.
b) graze on whatever you can find in a 10-metre radius without paying too much attention to what it is.
c) raid the glove box or desk drawer where you've hidden your emergency stash of jelly beans and Monster Munch.
d) scarf down your body weight in cereal bars and smoothies; you may be grumpy but you're on a diet, damnit.
e) eat your normal dinner, then raid the cupboards and fridge before bed, devouring your entire day's calorie count in a single sitting.

**2. You're out for dinner with your mates. Do you:**

a) order the shared starters with extra garlic mozzarella bread for everyone – you're all out together and what's a little bit of melted mozza between mates.
b) realize you've eaten more than your fair share of the bread basket before your starter has even arrived.
c) ignore the fact you're not hungry and order as much as everyone else anyway; those peanuts and crisps you scoffed while you were getting ready have filled you up temporarily, but it's a night out.
d) order the lowest-calorie dish on the menu and ask for the dressing on the side.
e) build up to a crescendo, hoovering up your starter and main before polishing off your dessert and everyone else's leftovers in one fell swoop.

**3. You've had a huge argument with him indoors while out shopping. Do you:**

a) head to the nearest McDonald's, making sure you order the largest portions available, plus a cheeseburger chaser and a McFlurry for pudding.

b) eat six packets of the kids' crisps when you get home before you've even taken your shoes off.

c) eat the final box of chocolates you've been hiding in the cupboard since Christmas, then dispose of the evidence before he gets home.

d) treat yourself to a huge fruit salad on the way home and prepare some sweet potato fries with roasted chicken breast for dinner.

e) wait at home until he gets back, have it out, have some make-up sex, then order a big curry for you both to celebrate.

**4. You're going on holiday tomorrow morning and you've realized you've got 300 euros more spending money than you thought. Do you:**

a) start the holiday early: make yourself a cocktail and crack out the cheese and biscuits or the Percy Pigs you were saving for the journey.

b) worry whether you'll still fit into your bikini after realizing you've absentmindedly finished a packet of chocolate digestives while you were packing.

c) buy and hide even more sweets and chocolate in your suitcase – you can afford it, after all.

d) splash out on extra goji berries and unsalted nuts for the plane journey.

e) put at least 100 euros aside for eats on the way back from nights out when you get there.

**5. You've had to cancel a planned anniversary meal with your bloke because you have to work late. Do you:**

a) cheer yourself up with treats from the office vending machine – if you're here for the long haul, you might as well try the different varieties of Tuc biscuits and Lucozade you've been eyeing up for weeks.

b) crack through the boiled sweets on your colleague's desk, finishing them before you've realized, and leave a Post-it note promising to replace them in the morning.

c) nip out for a portion of chips, hiding them in your drawer to eat them over the course of the next two hours finishing your presentation.

d) eat the roast vegetable, couscous and hummus wrap you left in the fridge at work for tomorrow's lunch.

e) promise yourself a pizza whenever you finally get out.

**6. You're preparing a Sunday roast for your family. Do you:**

a) gorge while you're preparing and cooking it – you need to make sure it all tastes good, after all.

b) absentmindedly nibble as you cook, from chopped raw carrots to dipping potatoes in the gravy, so that you're not hungry by the time you sit down, having eaten practically a whole meal while you've been cooking.

c) make sure you carve the chicken out of sight so you can eat your favourite bits as you go without having to share them with everyone else.

d) make sure some chicken breast is set aside for you and boil yourself some potatoes instead of eating the roasted ones.

e) eat a rabbit-sized portion round the table but raid the fridge in the wee small hours, dipping cold roasties in gravy.

**7. Your best friend calls on a Tuesday night to tell you she's just got engaged and wants to celebrate. Do you:**

a) turn up at her place within ten minutes bearing a large stuffed-crust Hawaiian, some Percy Pigs, Ferrero Rocher and Prosecco.

b) persuade her to check out the new cocktail bar in town and cruise up and down the bar eating all the free nuts while she talks wedding-dress designs.

c) make yourself a quick bowl of the Super Noodles you keep hidden at the back of the cupboard before heading over to hers – you need to line your stomach, after all, as this could be a big night.

d) tell her you'll stay out for a spritzer or two but need to quickly finish your steamed fish and roasted vegetable salad before you head over.

e) go all out – she's been waiting for a proposal for months – and treat her to a kebab on the way home to secure your bridesmaid role.

**8. Your niece confides in you that she hates school and doesn't have many friends. Do you:**

a) cheer her up with some solid aunty advice and some cream cakes for both of you.

b) realize you've eaten all the crisps you were supposed to be sharing while nodding sympathetically as she tells you her woes.

c) eat five biscuits in a row when you pop out to the kitchen to make you both a drink, feeling stressed out at the thought of her being bullied.

d) nibble thoughtfully on some vegetable crudités, while reminding her school won't last forever and soon it'll all be a distant memory.

e) put a brave face on it but worry your way through a tube of Pringles later when she's gone.

## 9. Your car breaks down on the way to meet a friend you haven't seen for years. Do you:

a) cry and eat snacks while you wait for the AA man – thank goodness you stopped off at the service station and got some treats to last you the journey.
b) suddenly realize half an hour later that you've eaten a whole bag of Minstrels while counting cars and looking out for the AA man.
c) make sure you've eaten the sandwich, Minstrels and crisps on the back seat and disposed of the evidence before the AA man arrives.
d) thank your lucky stars you bought your wholemeal pitta, falafel and tzatziki – you'd have been famished waiting so long without eating.
e) focus your thoughts on getting there eventually and enjoying the takeaway you've got planned for tonight.

## 10. You've broken your wrist falling over on a night out. Do you:

a) gain 4lb while in plaster – you're upset and depressed and fresh scones make everything better.
b) wonder why you've gained 4lb – until you realize the cupboards are bare and you've managed to cook and eat the entire contents of your kitchen with one hand.
c) figure out a way to keep a packet of Starburst hidden in your sling to keep you going while you recover.
d) stop buying bananas and opt for boxed fruit salad as you can't peel anything with one hand.

e) eat as little as possible during the day as only being able to use one hand is annoying, but make up for it when you take the sling off for a bit in the evening.

## If you answered mostly As:

## EMOTIONAL EATER

I feel your pain. You're an emotional eater. Whether you're happy, sad, angry or bored, whatever emotion you feel, you can find an excuse to eat to either make you feel better, pass the time, relieve the boredom or compound the misery. Take it from one emotional eater who learned the hard way: as long as you keep linking your emotions to food, you'll always have a battle on your hands. It's not an impossible cycle to break though. You need to start with baby steps to break the relationship. Next time you contemplate reaching for the biscuit barrel or takeaway menu to celebrate or commiserate, make yourself wait half an hour, or an hour if you can. If you still feel the same afterwards, allow yourself something small, or better still give yourself a treat that isn't calorie related. Book a massage, waste half an hour watching funny videos on YouTube, call a mate for a long overdue natter, run yourself a bath or paint your nails. Whatever you do, try and give yourself a treat to celebrate that isn't based on food. It'll be hard to begin with, but the more times you do it, the closer you'll come to breaking the cycle.

## If you answered mostly Bs:

## MINDLESS MUNCHER

You're a mindless eater. You've got what I like to call 'Cousin It' hands, which means they wander around of their own free will like you're not actually in control of them. You've a task and a half on your mitts, because most of the time you don't even realize what you're doing when your hand is feeding your face. We've all been there: you reach into the crisp bag or the biscuit barrel only to find it empty, but you can't remember finishing them. Being a mindless eater means you can consume a huge proportion of your daily calories without even tasting them or realizing you're doing it. Most people eat mindlessly when they're in the cinema watching a movie and eating popcorn, but you do it all the time. If you're a mindless eater, first of all you need to ensure the snacks you have on hand are healthy. Make sure you have plenty of fresh fruit and vegetables cut up and ready to snack on. Keep bags of seeds and nuts in the glove compartment of your car, your office desk and your handbag, so you're not tempted by the vending machine. And when you're eating, don't multitask – concentrate on the meal at hand and prioritize that above everything else. Mindless eaters munch more calories because they eat while they're reading, watching TV, doing the ironing or sending emails. Sit at the table for every meal and snack if you can. Stop eating in addition to doing something else, and then your brain and body will start to recognize the cues it gets as you start to fill up. You'll taste your food properly and find you stop eating as much, as you only eat until you're full.

*If you answered mostly Cs:*

## STEALTH SCRANNER

Come the apocalypse you'll be fine, because you've got food squirrelled away everywhere. You're a stealth eater – you've probably already fashioned a wine gum into a bookmark for this book. You're never far away from food and no doubt you've got hidden stashes of Werther's, Minstrels, biscuits, crisps and other sweets in your glove box, your desk drawers, your handbag, even your coat pockets. You probably consume a lot in secret, which won't do your waistline any good. Having a secret stash is no bad thing; I have them all over the place. But make sure the stash is healthy. If you've hidden healthy foods like fruit or nuts in place of your usual stodge, you can still satisfy the stealth-scranner element of your personality while protecting your waistline.

*If you answered mostly Ds:*

## HEALTHY HOGGER

You're trying so hard, aren't you? You think you're doing the right thing with your hummus and smoothies, your pittas and falafel, but your approach to dieting is scattergun. Whichever way you cut it, you're eating a lot of processed foods. Foods labelled 'low in fat' are often high in sugar. You're obsessed with healthy statements on packaging, but how much do you know about what really constitutes a balanced diet? The cereal bars you eat have a very high sugar content, so just because they're labelled 'made from oats' or 'contains real fruit', don't be fooled into thinking you're doing your waistline a favour. If you think you eat healthily but never lose weight, this could be the reason why. Educate yourself about the major food groups and which ones constitute a balanced diet. Try focusing more on fruit and vegetables and unprocessed foods. Pack your diet with vegetable crudités and fresh fruit salads, and instead of buying falafels and processed salads, make your own from scratch – they'll be free of additives and much more healthy and nutritious.

*If you answered mostly Es:*

## NIGHT-TIME NOSHER

You might appear to have a normal balanced diet, but it's likely you're consuming around a third of your daily food intake after dark. Night-time nibblers can develop the habit intentionally, or they may be too busy to eat properly during the day. Every time my weight has yo-yoed in the past it's been down to night-time nibbling. I'd follow my diet during the day but would find myself tempted by the bright lights of the fridge in the evenings. If you cut down your calorie intake too much during the day, your body goes into hunger mode and starts sending off powerful cravings in the evening, which is when your metabolism naturally starts to slow down. We tend to pay more attention to cravings at night because we're not so distracted by work, kids or chores and so hunger pangs always feel more intense. The worst thing you can do if you're trying to lose weight is to fill your tummy as your metabolism is slowing down in the evening – you'll retain more fat because your cells need less energy to do their job. Give yourself a cut-off point in the evening by which you want to have eaten all your meals. Make it realistic, though: if you're usually still chucking food down your neck at 10 p.m., move your cut-off to 9 p.m. to start off with, then reduce it by half an hour every week from then on, so that eventually you've finished eating by 7 p.m. and can give that poor metabolism of yours a proper well-earned rest.

## THREE

# Figure Out Your X-Factors – Stress, Genes and Your Body Type

I didn't need a genius to tell me I was an emotional eater. I think I'd always known it but figured it didn't really matter that much 'why' I ate. I thought what mattered was that I stopped eating as much in volume, stopped eating rubbish and started eating better and healthier foods.

I had 'diets' I would stick to for a while and I would lose weight, but I'd always gain it back again. I remember trying Slim Fast as a teenager and being delighted that I lost 10lb on it. I raved about it for years to anyone who'd listen – despite the fact that within three months of coming off it I'd gained 12lb. You see, that's the problem with diets: if they are effective in the short term, we forget that for us they didn't work in the long term.

My mate Sandra lost a stone on the 5:2 diet after she was invited to the wedding of her ex-boyfriend. She wanted to show him what he was missing out on. She looked amazing for about twelve weeks before she gained back all the weight and then some. She was a bit bothered, but still raved about her 'fasting' diet because it had helped her lose weight for a moment in time and look great – and she knew she could do it again if she needed to. (Incidentally, the ex came on to her at the wedding: she turned him down, but it put a smile on her face for months afterwards and gave her the confidence to join a dating website.)

But what if I told you that falling off the diet wagon might not be entirely to blame for your perennial battle with the bulge? What if there were other factors, other villains at work, sneaking about behind the scenes, derailing your best intentions and efforts to lose weight and keep it off for good? Villains you can't see or feel, let alone have the power to stop.

# Stress

What if I told you your boss was to blame? Or if I said your mortgage company increasing the rates on your borrowing was to blame? What if I told you your kids were to blame? They all are. They may not be the ones making you go back for seconds, but whatever is contributing to your stress levels has to take some of the blame for the size of your behind. The evidence of the relationship between hormones, stress and weight gain could fill the *Yellow Pages*; but if you're a stressy Sally, the chances are your emotional state is doing more harm to your waistline than a cheeky chicken shish kebab.

Stress kicks at you from all angles. When we're too pressured to prepare ourselves a decent healthy meal, we tend to resort to fast food, as it's quick, easy and familiar, as well as usually processed and full of junk. The times when you feel like you've got too much on your metaphorical plate are the times you pay the least attention to what you're putting on your actual plate. When we're stressed, a healthy, balanced diet is usually the first thing out the window and a bottle of wine is usually the first thing into the fridge.

Inevitably, what you eat is going to have an effect on your waistline, but in addition to taking less care about *what* we eat when we're stressed, the hormones raging around your system *when* we're stressed can have an actual physical effect on your waistline. In short, what you eat will make you fat, but so will how you feel.

When you're coping with stress, your body produces continuously high levels of the hormone cortisol, which under normal circumstances has a gentle pattern of ups and down through the day (highest in the early morning and lowest around midnight). Cortisol does many useful things in the body, including boosting blood sugar and energy levels, controlling blood pressure and regulating the digestive and immune systems. These are all important functions if you're to get through a bout of stress. But stress doesn't come in bouts anymore; it's an entirely different creature to what it was when humans first evolved. As you'll know if you suffer from stress, these days it's pretty continuous.

Imagine you're living in a cave thousands of years ago and you're attacked by a sabre-toothed tiger. Your stress levels would go through the roof and you'd need that initial burst of energy and adrenaline and follow-up dose of cortisol in order to defend your cave and open a can of whoop-ass on his furry behind. But when you feel stressed out all the time, your stress and cortisol levels are higher than they should be for longer than they should be, and your body is fooled into thinking it's using a lot of energy when it's not. The end result can be an increase in appetite, because your mind thinks you need extra energy.

As if that weren't enough, there's some evidence that cortisol can also affect *where* you put on weight. Some studies have shown that stress and elevated cortisol levels tend to mean you'll gain girth in the abdominal area, rather than in the hips. Ever known someone who's not expecting but has a big fat round pregnant-looking belly? If you give it a poke, it'll be hard – not soft like normal pudgy fat feels. This fatty build-up is referred to as 'toxic fat'. And toxic fat is strongly related to all sorts of heart and lung diseases. So you could be getting ill as well as fat unless you get those stressors in your life in check. Either way, stress is not the dieter's friend.

We all think we know what stress is and how it manifests itself. I used to think the same. But the fact is your body can start to suffer from the physical symptoms of stress way before your brain is aware of it. Just because you don't 'feel' stressed doesn't mean you're living in a Zen-like state and your stress hormones and cortisol levels are perfectly in balance.

I ask myself the questions below every few weeks to see how my stress levels are faring. If you can answer 'Yes' or even 'Hell, yeah!' to more than four of these questions, the chances are your stress levels are too high, and that means they may be contributing to your waistline and inhibiting your chances of sticking to a healthy diet and getting closer to your target weight.

**In the last fortnight have you:**
1. felt annoyed or upset by people's behaviour or trivial events?
2. felt impatient but struggled to put your finger on why?
3. found yourself feeling like you can't cope?
4. worried about whether you're a failure?
5. struggled to make decisions, either at home or at work?
6. started finding friends and your job boring for no good reason?
7. suffered with feelings of loneliness and abandonment, like you've got no one to talk to about how you really feel?
8. found it difficult to concentrate?
9. worried about how much you've got on your plate?

10. felt depressed or anxious?
11. experienced uncharacteristic aggressive feelings towards friends, family or colleagues?
12. felt bored and lacked drive?
13. started drinking, eating or smoking more?
14. started having more or less sex than normal with your partner?
15. found yourself overwhelmed with emotion at weird times to the point you felt like crying?
16. struggled to fall or stay asleep and felt exhausted all the time?
17. suffered from any of the following more frequently: back and neck pain, headaches, muscular aches and pains, muscular spasms and cramps, constipation, diarrhoea, loss of appetite, heartburn, in-digestion or nausea?
18. do you find yourself doing two or more of the following: biting your nails, clenching your fists, drumming your fingers, grinding your teeth, hunching your shoulders, tapping your feet?

You can do something about your stress levels, even if you can't tackle the cause of them. Over time you can train your mind to react differently to stress, to not let it get to you. Your kids are going to answer you back, him indoors is going to forget your anniversary and you'll never find anything to wear for your work Christmas do. These are irrefutable facts of life. You can't change any of those certainties, but you can change how you react to them.

# Genes

But while there's hope for your stress levels, there's another X-Factor you can't fix: your genes. Show me one overweight person who hasn't blamed their size on their genetic make-up. But while we've all used it as an excuse at some point, there's a grain of truth in there somewhere.

There *are* genes that are responsible for our weight: genes that make us hold onto fat for longer and slow down our metabolism; genes that inhibit our brains from telling us we're full; genes that make us prone to becoming easily addicted to things. Put simply, if you're big, the chances are you've got at least one fat gene, maybe more, which is making weight harder to shift and most likely easier to gain. These genes can lie dormant in even the slinkiest of mares and can be activated by environmental factors, like what you eat when you're growing up or which chemicals you get exposed to, but either way, once they're activated, you're in trouble. If you're big, there's every chance your genes loaded the gun and environmental factors pulled the trigger.

If you take a group of obese people and compare them with a group of people who are slender, many more of the first group will possess one or more fat genes linked with higher body weight, sure as Creme Eggs are Creme Eggs. That's just the way it is.

The study of the relationship between genetics and weight is going to explode in the next few years and anyone who doesn't believe fat genes exist is going to end up eating a large piece of humble pie. In the same way that we're targeting the genes that cause cancer at the moment and trying to isolate them so we can switch them off, at some point in the future we'll have made the scientific advances that'll mean we can isolate the fat genes and inhibit them, saving the NHS billions a year spent tackling obesity and related illnesses. I don't need to tell you how rich that's going to make the scientist that manages to do it.

But what, you may ask, has caused the explosion in obesity in the last few decades? Why now? Weight may have a significant genetic element, but surely us all getting fatter can't be down to DNA?

Well, yes and no. Of course there hasn't been an epidemic of big-belly gene mutations in just the last few decades – evolution doesn't work like that – but what we can say for sure is that never in the history of humankind have we been so swamped with such a huge amount of easily available food to wrap our gnashers around. Basically, we've grown greedy and our waistlines have expanded as a result. And while our genes are our genes and the environment is the environment, the two of those things interact in the most intimate and sinister way to make us eat more and more.

Take for example the FTO gene – those of us with two high-risk copies of the gene (thanks, Mum and Dad!) are 70 per cent more likely to become obese than those with low-risk genes. Seventy per cent! Those are great odds at a bookie's. In evolutionary terms, back in the day, the very FTO mutations that make us fat and unhealthy now were necessary and even life-saving, because they motivated us to go and spear a woolly mammoth when we were on the verge of starvation and there was barely enough food to survive. The gene might also have helped us pile on the pounds quicker in the summer so we could survive through the harsher winters.

But in the modern world, the FTO gene that once helped us stay alive is pretty useless, because food is no longer scarce, so we don't need our genes to protect us and keep us alive. It's the same principle as with our cortisol levels. When we were evolving we needed these genes, but now they're no longer vital, they've started to do more damage than good. If you've got a weight-gaining version of FTO, you're going to have a higher level of the hunger hormone ghrelin and you're going to find fatty foods more tempting. In short, with food everywhere, you're going to have a hard time of it and not just because you may be weak-willed.

It's not all doom and gloom, though. Think of people with fat genes (and there are many genes that affect weight, not just FTO), as the survivors of this world. We'd have been the ones running the show if we were still living in the Stone Age. As it is, we have to work way harder than the average person does to stay slim. I've got more than my fair share of fat genes and as a result I'm always hungrier than my skinny mates, I can't tell as easily when I'm full, which means I'm liable to overeat unless I'm constantly vigilant, and as if things weren't bad enough, I have to exercise more willpower and self-control to say no to biccies because the hormones in my body think I need them.

I was always the one asking for the dessert menu if I went out with the girls, whereas most of them have the motivation to just opt for a coffee after dinner. I was also the minesweeper finishing off their final couple of chips or griddled asparagus. The difference is that now I recognize I want to do it, and so most of the time I'm able to steel myself not to give in to temptation. Learning about the roles of genetics and stress in my own weight battle has made me more aware of the choices I am making and the reactions I have to food. Once I was aware of these factors I could start to act on them and make changes.

So there you have it. If I've ranted on a bit about the extra struggle you're going to face if you were born with unlucky genes, don't get too glum: I'm just trying to redress the balance for all those times you've thought that it's 100 per cent your own fault that you're bigger than your mates and can't shake your addiction to donuts.

I hate those skinny people who say: 'Just lose weight, stop eating crap, stop overeating, do some exercise . . .' It's all well and good to say that if you're born skinny. Those people will never know what it's like to battle their genes. When I was a big bird and was trolled online, my Twitter bullies thought I was fat because I was a lazy, greedy slob. I know I was to some extent; but my genes won't ever be like Abbey Clancy's. A lot of my size was my fault, but not all of it. Genes aren't the only reason you can't get into your jeans; but this is an area of emerging research, and one day we'll know more about genetics and their relationship to weight and which specific diet and exercise approach is best suited for you and your genetic make-up. You'll be given more of a break when you bemoan your fat genes because people will know they exist.

But while you can't change your genes, and they can be partly blamed for your booty, along with your stress hormones, you've got to take your portion of the blame too. Let's say, for the sake of argument, that at least 50 per cent of your weight is still determined by what you do have control over, for example, what you eat and how much you move around. You can blame your genes all you like – God knows I did for long enough – but at the end of the day, while they might be partly responsible for your dress size, they're not the only culprit.

# Work With Your Body, Not Against It

I hid behind my excuse of being big-boned for decades, but just like blaming genetics, it turns out it wasn't a complete lie. In addition to my genes, my body type didn't do me any favours.

Knowing what kind of eater you are is only half the battle. Knowing your body type will help you set goals that are realistic and help you on the way to becoming the best version of yourself you can be. There's no point me longing to be a waif when I'm naturally curvy – I'd die trying. The three main body types are known as endomorph, ectomorph and mesomorph. In plain English, that's fat retainers, skinny Minnies and athletic birds. There are very few women who are a single body type; most of us are a mixture and will be one body type predominantly but with slight characteristics of another. I'm an endomorph, a fat retainer, with small tendencies towards a mesomorph. It takes me ages to lose weight, but I can gain 4lb to 6lb overnight if I fall off the wagon. But when I lost the fat coat I'd worn for years, I realized I had quite an athletic frame under all that blubber. Recognizing your body type and knowing the rate at which you gain and store fat makes it easier to develop a workout plan specifically to suit your needs and targets.

As Penny says in *Dirty Dancing*, 'God wouldn't have given you maracas if he didn't want you to shake 'em.' There's no point wishing you were a 6ft-tall Amazonian goddess if you're 5ft 3in and flat-chested. Be realistic about what your expectations are: you're trying to lose weight, remember, not become a completely different person. By the end of your journey you should be able to look yourself in the mirror and admit you're the very best version of yourself that you can be. That's your number one priority. It certainly was mine.

I'll never be the petite, elfin, Hepburn-esque beauty I longed to be in my teens – not with my naturally wide hips and size-7 feet. But I can be curvy and statuesque, the best version of myself I can be. Knowing your body type will help you set realistic goals and manage realistic expectations.

## YOU'RE AN ENDOMORPH/FAT RETAINER IF:

- you've got wider hips than shoulders
- you gain weight easily but find losing it hard
- any weight you gain settles around your middle: hips, thighs, bum, tum
- you tire easily and are prone to fatigue
- you find it hard to maintain weight-loss

*Best diet*

When you're trying to lose weight, hunger can be an endomorph's biggest issue, so you need to look for foods that have a low energy density – i.e. foods that are going to fill you up but not out. Lean protein, like chicken, fish and prawns, helps curb your appetite by making you feel fuller for longer. Team it with lots of high-fibre, water-filled foods that fill up your stomach, like soups, and non-starchy veg and you'll go some way to curbing the hunger that controls most of your food choices.

## YOU'RE AN ECTOMORPH/SKINNY MINNIE IF:

- you've got long arms and legs in proportion to a shorter body
- you've got a small chest and bum
- you go straight up and down without going in anywhere

- you can be prone to bouts of hyperactivity
- you find it hard to build muscle

*Best diet*

You were probably able to eat loads of sweets as a kid without gaining any weight, but older ectomorphs can pile on love handles if they don't keep refined carbs in check. Do yourself a favour by ditching the sugar and switching to a low glycaemic index (low GI) diet with modest amounts of slow-releasing carbs: root veg, sweet potatoes and the occasional skin-on spud, firm bananas, berries and quinoa.

## YOU'RE A MESOMORPH/ATHLETIC BIRD IF:

- you're wider at the shoulders than the hips
- you're naturally strong
- you've got broad, square shoulders
- your body responds to exercise when you can be bothered to do it
- you've got poor flexibility and struggle to touch your toes

*Best diet*

You respond well to a balanced diet with plenty of lean protein. Good fats like avocados, nuts and coconut oil along with plenty of veg, some fruit and some slow-releasing carbs (root veg, sweet potatoes and the occasional skin-on spud, firm bananas, berries and quinoa) should all be on your 'to eat' list. With the right exercise, your body puts on muscle pretty much whatever you feed it, but you still need to maintain a healthy balance for optimal health. You are more able than other body types to counteract a fall off the diet wagon as long as you keep working out, but don't use this as an excuse to eat processed rubbish.

# Homework

Once you know more about the body you've got to work with, you get the fun job of choosing your thinspiration. Now this isn't something to rush into lightly. I played with Cheryl Cole, JLo and Halle Berry (not literally), before setting my sights on Raquel Welch. She became the screensaver on my iPad, the wallpaper on my phone; I carried pictures of her in my wallet, stuck them to my fridge and had her poster on my wall. I wrote her measurements down in every notebook I had and they were highlighted on every page of my food diary.

I read every interview with her I could find and despite being 4,000 miles away in Tinseltown, Raquel came with me on my weight-loss journey and was right beside me every step of the way. I'd try and make decisions about what I ate as if I was her. At restaurants I'd think, 'What would Raquel order?' When I was working out I'd think, 'Raquel would push herself harder', and it'd give me the encouragement I needed to try that little bit harder. I know I'm a little bit of an obsessive, but she became like my imaginary friend. Willing me on every day. Smiling at me from the fridge door in her bikini, reminding me that I too could have a body like hers one day. I too could look hot in a Stone Age bikini. Over the course of seven months in 2011, Raquel and I formed a bond which can never be broken. We shared together, suffered together and succeeded together. Raquel and Josie: sisters in arms.

Finding the right thinspiration for your body type will motivate you and put a smile on your face when you don't think you can push yourself any harder.

# FOUR

# Find Your Motivation

As I've said before, successful dieting is mostly about the mind. You need the willpower to stick to your new healthy eating plan when times get hard and you really, really want to munch your way through a packet of chocolate biccies. One way to keep motivated is to remember your wake-up call – that moment when you realized you had to change. Mine came in the form of massive public humiliation.

Until I lost weight for good in 2012, I'd been thin twice in my life. Both times after break-ups. Every woman I know, no matter what size, has put themselves on two diets in their lives: the Atkins Diet and the Heartbreak Diet. Breaking up with someone, whether it's your choice or not, is a sure-fire way to drop a few dress sizes.

The first time Cupid helped out my waistline was when I split up with my first love, Kevin – I was twenty-two years old and thought he was Mr Forever After when really he was Mr Having Sex With Tons Of Other Women Behind My Back. He may have broken my heart emotionally, but physically he probably did it a favour, as I lost 3 stone with all the stress, heartbreak and humiliation. Of course, I soon piled it back on, and more.

The second time was after I came out of the *Big Brother* house. I'd started seeing John James Parton while I was in the house, and when the show ended and I won, I was thrust into the limelight as Josie Gibson, winner of *Big Brother* and one half of what everyone presumed was a fake couple because he was very good-looking and I was obese. I should have seen the writing on the wall when people tried to make us look as different as they could at every photo shoot we did. He'd be the hot one in jeans with a bit of he-vage on show and I'd be the one in the background looking like his mum in floaty cover-ups with middle-aged beads around my fat wrists and double chin.

People genuinely didn't believe someone who looked like me could pull someone who looked like him. Looking back, I'm not sure I believed it either. We split up, after seven miserable months together, in January 2011, and he started dating a size-8 model within weeks. That summer I was papped stuffing my face in Marbella in a bikini, not realizing my belly was hanging over my waistband and onto my chunky thighs. He retweeted the hideous picture of me, laughing about it with his friends and followers on Twitter. I was put right off my kebabs, replaced meals with fags and was soon on my way to being a size 12. That's what embarrassment and a broken heart does for you.

Then I met my Lukey Sanwo, a beautiful 6ft 4in prince. I did what we all do in the first throes of love – apart from go on the pill – I gained weight. The Heartbreak Diet I'd been on since splitting up with John fell by the wayside and was soon replaced with dinners out, takeaways in and nights down the pub with my new love.

You see, that's the thing about dieting after a break-up: you might end up with an empty heart and tum, but as soon as one is filled, the other one invariably is too. Needless to say I'd gone up to a size 14 by the time Luke asked me to marry him in January 2012, during a romantic night cruise on the River Thames. And when we decided to celebrate our engagement with my friends and family down in Bristol a month later, I was almost a size 16 again.

At 5ft 11in, overweight and with really high foot arches, I don't often wear heels. Back then I was more a flats and maxi dress kind of girl. Everyone who's big knows that trying to balance the extra timber in heels is a task and a half, but my engagement party was a special night. Or at least it was until I broke my ankle falling off my skyscraper heels. Nearly 14 stone landed on my ankle bone the wrong way, when I'd gone out for a ciggie and snapped it in two.

To say I was at a pretty low ebb over the next few weeks would be putting it mildly. Lukey and I were in the first throes of our romance. I was used to him taking me from behind; now he was taking me to the bog – and that's not a euphemism. We were in the middle of moving from London down to Bristol to start a new life together, and there I was, ordering him around, telling him what to pack in each box, sending him down the shop for sweets and treats and generally being a pain in his pert behind, while he was helping me wipe mine. I sat there cursing my stupidity, my cast and my weight, which was making it impossible for me to move around. Bearing nearly 14 stone on two legs is hard enough; doing it on one while using a set of crutches is completely exhausting.

Two months later, I'd gained even more weight and was suffering from insomnia and depression, having spent almost all my time trapped in my sixth-floor redbrick tower, moaning that Lukey had bought the wrong kind of biscuits and had eaten the last bit of Viennetta before checking with me. I was like Rapunzel with a penchant for junk food, but my hair extensions weren't as long or of as much use.

The cast finally came off two months later (don't even get me started on how hairy and smelly my pegleg was). But with my mobility restored, my legs waxed and a new pedicure, I decided to go to Ibiza for a few days to clear the depressive fog I'd been lost in and let Lukey handle the rest of the move. I was close to 16 stone and a size 20, but thought a bit of sun would cheer me up; besides, people look thinner with a tan, or so I thought. I was feeling really sorry for myself and my default setting was to find comfort in food and alcohol – starting with a dirty great plate of chips and a gorgeous bottle of cold crisp rosé the day after I arrived. But while I obliviously supped my vino and scoffed my deep-fried spuds, I don't need to tell you muckers what happened next.

When *those* bikini pictures appeared everywhere, I didn't leave the house for four weeks. The first morning the pictures came out, I remember getting a call from my agent telling me I'd made it into the big league. I thought some foreign executive had asked to see my show reel, or I'd been cherry-picked for a new presenting gig somewhere exciting. Instead he told me I'd made newspaper headlines and magazine covers all over the world because I'd been papped in my pink two-piece on my holiday in Ibiza. He thought any publicity was good publicity.

Within days everyone was mocking me, from New Zealand to New York. One morning I woke up to over 100 tweets directed at me. I took a deep breath and started checking through the comments. I'd scrolled down the first twenty of them before tears started to prick my eyes. The pictures had appeared in the *National Enquirer* in America and it seemed the world wanted to tell me I was obese, disgusting and deserved to die. There were a couple of blokes offering to pay me to fly over and sit on them – every cloud has a silver lining and all that. But the rest of them had me in floods of tears and cursing myself before I'd even got out of bed or put the kettle on. 'Looks Like Shamu Made It To Land' laughed an

American blog. '*Quelle Horreur!*' echoed a French one. Now I don't speak the lingo, but I'm pretty sure that's not complimentary. I was called a 'fat and ugly c*nt' every single day on Twitter and people went out of their way to tell me how disgusting I was. The pictures were used in every newspaper in the UK and in magazines all over the globe.

And while the negative press attention was new to me, so was the trolling. You see, despite being big, I'd never been bullied at school. Maybe I was left alone because I was always pretty hard; but whatever the reason, I preferred to knock people out with a punchline rather than a punch when they joked about my weight. But as I now learned, bullies aren't made like they used to be. These days, you can't just offer them out and come away with your pride intact – they've got laptops and fake IDs to hide behind. I drove myself mad trying to answer back to the hundreds of faceless, nameless and gutless cowards who'd spend hours abusing me from the safety of their computer screens.

I'd sit for days, not showering, staring at my four walls and sucking my thumb – a habit I've never been able to break – before refreshing Twitter to see what other names I'd been called. I was helpless and couldn't do anything but take it. Answering back gave them the validation they were after; once they'd got my attention, the trolls' insults would get worse and come thicker and faster. Call me a fat disgusting mess once and I'll laugh it off and call you a liar. Call me a fat disgusting mess hundreds of times a day and I'll start to believe you.

I know I looked a state (if you're size 20, it's never advisable to wear a two-piece, let alone run in one), but the backlash was vicious and vitriolic. I'd never been attacked so remorselessly by so many complete strangers. The depression and self-loathing that set in left me under the darkest cloud I'd ever known.

I knew I was a big girl, but until those pictures appeared I'd always thought my boat race was all right. I used to joke with my mates that they were lucky their blokes didn't run off with me. I knew I was never going to be Miss World – but having complete strangers call you a fat munter in eight or nine different languages every day? That's going to wear down even the most confident mucker.

I kept trying to put a brave face on it, but I was feeling lower than I had in years. I stopped having sex with Lukey and started pushing him away. I couldn't stand him touching me. Despite him telling me he still found me sexy and didn't care what anyone else said, I didn't believe him any more. How could it be true? I found out he was being bullied at work because of how disgusting I looked: they'd cut the pictures of me out of the papers, stuck them everywhere and called him a 'fatty fucker'. I tried to joke my way out of it, reminding people I hadn't met a man I couldn't laugh into bed, but with Lukey at work all day, I spent more time than is healthy monitoring what people were saying about me online, looking down at the rolls of fat and reaching for the Roast Beef Monster Munch for a quick fix.

You see, I was depressed and fixing the problem – dropping five dress sizes – seemed a daunting and impossible task. So instead of figuring out how to do it, I turned to the fridge, cupboards and takeaway menus to sate the emotional hunger and hurt. But when you're licking your finger and using it to scoop up the final few crumbs at the bottom of the biscuit barrel, the fear and torment kicks in again. The next minute you'll still be just as fat, but you'll have taken a step backwards thanks to McVitie's chocolate digestives – and to add insult to injury, there'll be no biscuits left in the house. Comfort eating might work while your jaws are masticating, but the minute you swallow you'll be that little bit lower, and fatter, than before.

Trying to explain this relationship to anyone who's never used food as an emotional crutch is impossible. But if you've ever reached for the confectionery counter to put a smile on your face, you'll understand how you can become enslaved to this Groundhog Day nightmare cycle of depression and bingeing. Depression and obesity are inextricably linked, and not just in my life.

A recent study published in the journal *Public Health Nutrition* found that people who ate junk food were over 50 per cent more likely to show signs of depression than people who didn't. And the clincher that proves my point? The more junk food the participants in the study ate, the more likely they were to be depressed.

Chicken or egg, egg or chicken? It doesn't matter which came first. If you're depressed and fat, who cares which one happened at the beginning? The fact is, the two things often come as a very dangerous pair. In my case, I'll never be able to establish which one came first. I was always big, with an appetite to match. But I remember being low and depressed from when I was a child. I know the junk food led to my feeling rubbish about myself, but that, in turn, led to consuming more food and even lower lows. It doesn't matter which way round this horrible roller coaster starts, because at the end of the day the results are much the same as riding Oblivion at Alton Towers but without the exhilaration – you soon end up in a deep, dark hole in the ground wondering how you got there and struggling to believe you'll ever find a way out.

When you think about it, the internal dialogue you have when all this is going on – the beating yourself up and telling yourself you're the crappiest person on earth – that actually *is* depression. Ever heard of the phrase 'depression is anger turned inward'? When you use food as an emotional crutch, you feel tired, sad, lonely, hopeless and thoroughly convinced that you're an incapable person destined to be trapped in your overweight shell. You have trouble getting up in the morning and getting to sleep at night. You don't follow through on things that you'd like to do because you have no faith in your ability to succeed. I'd wanted to lose weight plenty of times in my life, but I didn't believe I could do it and I didn't think I was worth the effort. I hated who I was but changing it seemed such a daunting and impossible task, it seemed much easier to just reach for the ginger nuts.

The regular black cloud of depression I was used to waking up under turned even darker and so did my thoughts. I always tried to see the funny side when I was teased about my weight. I had a long list of comebacks about being big. But now, even I couldn't see a funny side. I started receiving abusive text messages on my personal phone from a number I didn't recognize: there were people telling me I should stop eating for five minutes to buy a noose and hang myself. I was called a fat, disgusting, washed-up beached whale and told that every man who I'd ever slept with probably had to close his eyes to stop himself being sick. There were texts and tweets telling me I didn't deserve to live, that I was taking up too much air and too much space and should die. I spent hours reading and rereading them, over and over again, the words twisting like a knife. I'd read the same tweet ten times in a row trying to make sense of it or trying to find a meaning other than the literal one – that I should kill myself. I'd feel my eyes pricking with tears and would look away to compose myself, staring at the view from my sixth-floor balcony and wondering if they were right. Maybe I did deserve to die. Maybe I was taking up too much air and too much space. Maybe I was so disgusting I shouldn't exist any more.

Within hours, I found I couldn't take my eyes off the railings on my balcony. I'd go out for a cigarette and push and pull on them, wondering whether they'd take my weight if I tied on a noose, put it around my neck and jumped off. It would be a quick end, wouldn't it? A quick snap and the misery would be over. But what if the railings didn't take my weight and I fell from the sixth floor? I might have laughed if I hadn't felt so bleak and dark. There I was contemplating suicide and yet again my weight was standing in the way. I wasn't even sure I could kill myself because I was so fat I might just break the railings and end up six floors down in the bushes with another broken limb.

I spent the entire day while Luke was at work wondering whether my tormentors were right. Maybe I should be dead. Maybe I'd be thin in heaven. Left alone with my thoughts and Twitter, I spiralled into a deep misery which I only snapped out of the minute Luke put his key in the door. When he walked towards me and planted a kiss on my head, it reminded me of everything I had to live for. And everyone I owed my strength to. Everyone who knew and loved me, who'd have been heartbroken to know I let bullies get the better of me. What was I thinking? I'd never let anyone beat me in life before; why was I about to start now, just because of some pictures in the papers?

It was the kick up the arse I needed. I'd show them. Show them all. I'd start eating right and exercising. I'd develop my own diet. This diet would save my life. I would do it properly this time. I'd show them all who I really was, who I really could be. Who I should have been all my life. I called a personal trainer that night and booked him for the next two months.

You don't have to be a rocket scientist to know that sometimes you need a wake-up call to change your life. But mine was the most hurtful, humiliating and degrading experience of my life and drove me too close to suicide for comfort. My wake-up call was splashed all over the world's media and made some paparazzi very rich indeed; but if I'm being honest, there were plenty of other wake-up calls before then that I chose to ignore. So should I blame the paparazzi lurking on the beach or myself? What about the time I couldn't even do up the knee-high boots I tried on in Evans – in *Evans*! Or the time Candice, my best friend in the world, bought me a flight in a bi-plane for my eighteenth birthday. I'd had to starve myself for a month to lose nearly a stone to fit into the seat because I was too fat and heavy to qualify for the compulsory insurance.

I ignored my wake-up calls for years because it suited me, and I didn't know how to fix things even if I'd wanted to. If someone had waved a magic wand and I could have been thin overnight, I'd have bitten their hand off – and probably chewed it and swallowed it. But the bottom line was that I hated the thought of working out, dieting and changing my life more than I hated being fat, and until that equation changes you'll ignore every wake-up call you hear. I'm sure that while you've been reading these words, you've been thinking about the wake-up calls that have gone by and you've chosen to ignore.

That's fine, sister; I'm not here to judge. But, despite everything, I often think about how lucky I am that my wake-up call was just a set of pictures of me looking like Shamu the whale in a pink bikini plastered over the world's media, and not the heart attack or diabetes diagnosis that would have happened sooner or later. Seeing those pictures and experiencing that bullying was the boot up the bum I needed. I couldn't keep going the way I was. I was depressed; I hated myself; my insomnia and mental-health issues were both weight-related; I teared up almost every time I looked in the mirror; and I had spent years pushing every partner I had away because I was filled with self-loathing. Something had to give. I had to lose weight or die trying.

# Homework

Write down the last three wake-up calls you chose to ignore – and how they made you feel.

1. _____

   _____

   _____

2. _____

   _____

   _____

3. _____

   _____

   _____

When things get tough and you feel like giving up, you can look back at this page and remind yourself how you felt. Consider the fact that you're reading this book as a wake-up call in itself, and tell yourself you are ready to change from the inside out.

# FIVE

# Believe You're Worth It

When I decided to lose weight for good, the desperation I felt was like nothing I'd ever experienced. I used to lie in bed at night looking at my hands, wondering which finger I'd chop off if someone gave me the option of getting rid of a digit to lose a few pounds. I'd have sold my soul to be instantly thin. I wanted it more than I've ever wanted anything in my life – even more than the Sylvanian Families caravan I'd wanted when I was six and bugged Mum about for two years solid.

It felt so hopeless, like I was starting a journey I had no idea if I'd finish. Was I going to make it to my size-10 destination? Or – like every other time I'd tried to lose weight – would I end up right back at the beginning? The trepidation and terror I felt all the time at the thought my struggle might be in vain was overpowering. I might just be destined to be fat for good. After all, I'd never managed to lose weight and keep it off before – what would make this time any different? Why would it work now when every other time I'd failed miserably?

I started listening to all the voices in my head, both the ones telling me I could do it and the ones telling me I'd never make it. My confidence would either be sky-high or down in the dumps, never anywhere in between. I'd either hit training on a high and want to push myself to extremes, or I'd be on the verge of tears for the hour I was there trying to think of excuses to get out of it, even hoping I would sprain a limb so the workout could end. I was just wasting my personal trainer's time, my time and my money.

The feeling of despair is one of the most negative emotions you can feel on your weight-loss journey. You can channel other negative feelings into something more positive, but despair and hopelessness have no 'bright side'. When you're angry at yourself for getting fat, you can turn that into motivation for a workout. When you're upset that you got into this state, you can turn it into an emotional release – have a good cry and that will leave you feeling calmer and ready to keep going with your eating plan. But despair has no upside, no kernel of positivity you can glean from it and work with. It's empty and destructive.

The other problem with despair is that not only do you long for what you don't have, but you also begin to loathe and hate what you do have. The two feelings are inextricably linked. I longed to be slim and the more I longed for it, the more I grew to detest what I was. Every roll, every lump, every peel of cellulite and bulge of a bingo wing I had.

If you let despair own you, you'll be too busy hating what you've become, and blaming yourself for ignoring the problem for so long, to focus on now and the future. Being an Aquarian, I always try to look on the bright side. OK, I ignored my weight problem for the whole of my teenage years and most of my twenties, but I woke up to the truth eventually. Don't let despair keep you from focusing on the positives. Yes, you could have got here sooner, you could have lost weight ten, twenty or maybe even thirty years ago. But you're here now. So deal with your despair and focus on where you're heading, rather than where you've been.

# Sexy Selfie Time

Go and stand in front of the biggest mirror you have – a full-length one is perfect – and spend a few minutes looking at yourself. It's all right to notice all the bits you hate first – that's what we all do when we're big. But look past your thick waist and thighs, see more than your bingo wings, hips, fat wrists and double chin. Stand a little longer and see, I mean *really* see yourself, from every angle you can.

Find three things you like about yourself – trust me, when I first did this I was there for about half an hour trying to find one, let alone three – but the fact is, everyone's got their good bits. Whether you like your boobs, your nails, your eyes or your skin, it doesn't matter. It can be a look on your face, or a stance, or the way your hair falls down your back. What matters is that you stay in front of the mirror and stand and stare at yourself long enough to start to see yourself differently – admit that while there are things you need to change, there are also things that are just fine the way they are. Things you could learn to feel proud of.

Remember: this is your body. Your own amazing work of art. You're the designer. With knowledge, power and determination you can sculpt yourself into whatever you want to be. Don't think you've gone too far and there's no way back – that's a lazy excuse and you know it. Everything is reversible. The body you're walking around in is an amazing feat of engineering that *you're* in control of, something you can fix and change however you want. It doesn't matter what it looks like now; what matters is what it *will* look like – what you can transform it into.

## TAKE A PICTURE

Now, this is far and away one of the hardest things you're going to have to do, so take your time and make sure you do it properly. Strip down to your undercrackers and take two photos of yourself: one full frontal and one sideways on. I did this every week for the six months it took me to lose weight. If you're anything like I was, you'll have spent years refusing to let people take full-length pictures of you, so you'll probably hate it for the first few weeks. The thought of having to repeat the process every week will fill you with about as much excitement as the prospect of root canal treatment, but when you see things starting to change, you'll feel a million dollars and be glad you made yourself do it.

I promise you that in a month's time you'll get excited at the prospect of stripping off for the camera – it'll fast become the highlight of your week.

When I look back through my pictures and see the smile on my face the first time I realized I could look down and see my mimsy because my belly had shrunk, I'm so glad I had a camera there to document my disbelief and delight. Looking back and being able to physically see as well as measure how many inches I've lost off my belly fills me with pride.

## MEASURE YOURSELF

Now it's time to get your tape measure and scales out. I spent years refusing to have a set of scales in the house. I didn't want to know what I weighed and preferred to stay in ignorant bliss. But if you're ever going to face what you need to fix, you need to know the extent of the task ahead. Invest in a good set of scales and weigh yourself in pounds – they come off faster than kilos, so you'll feel like you're making better progress. Once a week, take a tape measure and measure your tum, hips, thighs, boobs and anything else you feel like measuring. Now weigh yourself. Write everything down in the back of a notebook; you'll need the front of it for your food diary.

Once you've written your first load of measurements down, I guarantee you'll be tempted to stray to the fridge or cupboards to try and find something to eat to make yourself feel better, but don't. Give yourself half an hour (an hour if you can) to absorb and process what you've just done. If you're still hungry afterwards, go ahead. Which brings me to your food diary.

## KEEP A FOOD DIARY

From now on, I want you to write down every morsel of food and drop of liquid that passes your lips. Everything – from nicking the kids' leftover toast crusts at breakfast to finishing off the last roaster left in the pan after Sunday lunch or the piece of cake in the office kitchen on a workmate's birthday. Don't cheat. As Mrs Anderson, my junior-school headmistress, used to say, 'You're only cheating yourself.' You can go old-school like I did and write it all in a notebook, or you can download an app to help you keep track; either is fine. What matters is that you document it. You'll realize how often you eat because you're bored, or stressed, or just because the food is in front of you, and that will help knock those bad habits on the head.

Studies have shown that slimmers who track their weightloss with photos and food diaries lose more weight than those who don't, sometimes up to twice as much. So get cracking, no matter how awkward you feel. We all have to start somewhere – remember every great shopping trip starts with a single step.

## FIND A POSITIVE AFFIRMATION

Once you've taken your picture and recorded your measurements, have a chat to yourself.* Find an encouraging phrase you're comfortable saying and repeat it a few times. I kept telling myself I could be a sexy mare. I told myself that almost every day for six months, each morning and evening looking in the mirror, and look at me now (except for first thing in the morning with no make-up on). You'll feel like a right tool the first few times you say it, but take your time, look yourself square in the eye and keep saying it until you really mean it.

Positive affirmations had as much of a part to play in my weight-loss journey as my workout routines, but in order for them to work, your affirmation has to be something you really believe and something you can realistically achieve. Telling myself I could do it and would be sexy one day gave way to me actually believing it. Sometimes self-belief can make all the difference. Look in the mirror, picture a nice healthy body shape and imagine you in it.

## SET TARGETS

Next, write down a list of your targets. Don't make them just about a number on the scales or your dream dress size – set some health and fitness targets too. Whether it's coming first in the parents' race at sports day, playing volleyball on the beach next summer or swimming in the sea when you next go on holiday, find realistic targets you can work towards. I wanted to be able to climb stairs

---

* Not too loudly or the neighbours will think you've lost it.

without getting out of breath and I wanted to be able to cycle from my house into the city of Bristol four miles away without breaking into a sweat. I wanted to climb a mountain in Switzerland. I wanted to wear a bodycon dress. I wanted to wear a two-piece on the beach and have people look at me for the right reasons, not the wrong ones. I also wanted to be a size 10 and 10 stone, but the numbers weren't my only motivation. I wanted to be able to carry my mates' kids when they got tired in the park without huffing and puffing and having to put them down. Having all-round targets means you're fighting on all fronts, but you've got lots of mini-victories in store too. I was able to scoop up my friend J's little boy in the park way before I got to my milestone weight, but it was still a victory I celebrated because it was a target I'd set right at the beginning.

# Homework

You've made it to the end of step 1, but before you skip merrily onto step 2, make sure you've done your homework.

Find out where your issues with food come from:

- Work out what kind of eater you are, so you can break the cycle before you fall back into bad habits. Find what will motivate you and remind yourself of it when you are tempted by junk food and the biscuit barrel.
- Take a picture of yourself, front and sideways on. Do this every week until you get to your target weight.
- Weigh and measure yourself and write down your measurements in your notebook. Do this once every week.

- Start a food diary and keep it going as you change your eating habits.
- Write down between five and ten realistic targets.
- Find a positive affirmation and repeat it to yourself – you *are* worth it and you *can* do this.

# STEP 2

# How to Eat Lots of Healthy Food *and* Lose Weight

# Introduction

Over the years I'd tried every short cut and quick fix imaginable in my decade-long battle with the bulge. Being a Gibson, if there was a way of doing something that wasn't completely above board, I'd find it. As girls do when they get to their teens – especially ones who'd been nine stone at nine years old – I started dabbling in diets, but healthy eating didn't come into it. To me, a balanced diet meant a bag of rhubarb and custard in one blazer pocket and a bag of Kola Kubes in the other.

I went through periods when I longed to be thin. I remember when the lad I fancied in my fifth year at secondary school said he'd be my boyfriend and have sex with me as long as I told no one. I thought it was our special romantic secret. In my head we were star-crossed lovers, but the reality was that he was OK with a bit of rumpy-pumpy with the class fattie, he just didn't want his mates to know he liked chubbers. I found out how he really felt when he started going out publicly with the gorgeous size-6 girl at school. I'd have given anything not to be his dirty little secret, to make him proud of me rather than ashamed.

I thought losing weight meant starving myself all day to the point of being light-headed and feeling sick, then scranning down six slices of white toast with butter before bed. I figured dieting was meant to be agony: shoving bland, boring foods down my neck, rather than lush, tasty, flavourful grub. I was sure to lose weight, so long as I had to either starve, cheat or better still both. Enter diet pills stage left.

I can say honest to God that there probably isn't a diet pill on the market – legal or illegal – that I haven't tried in my desperation to be thin. From slimming injections – bought from America on the internet – to diet pills that speed up your metabolism, suppress your appetite, speed up your heart rate, block fat, leave you constipated or incontinent, turn your wee green, give you heavier periods, irregular periods or insomnia, I've tried the lot. Some of them would work, or so I would think, but inevitably the minute I stopped taking them, I'd pile all the weight back on – and usually then some. You see, I was still eating rubbish, so I wasn't tackling the root cause of the problem.

I always wondered what it would be like to be thin. Everyone I knew who was a skinny Minnie seemed so happy. So sorted, perfect and complete. They all seemed to have the good jobs, the sexy blokes and the fab wardrobes, while I worked on a production line putting together tumble dryers or shredding paper for animal bedding, and sat at home watching MTV on my own in my jammies.

But instead of thinking about following a proper healthy balanced diet, which probably would have been the cheaper option as well as the smarter one, I threw good money after bad chasing a quick fix, a pipedream. I was one of those lazy dieters, the ones who think they're doing right and eating well but can't be bothered to read or research anything. They live by soundbites or headlines and never educate themselves properly. The ones who think all fats are bad and all carbs are the devil, that dieting shouldn't be fun and needs to be a slog. I used to cram my trolley full of granary bread, not realizing it's barely any better for you than white bread. I ate cereal bars, unaware that some of them contain more sugar than your recommended daily amount. I scoured the aisles for 'low fat' labels, not even considering that low-fat products can be high in sugar and calories. Heck, I even paid attention to calories, which now seems utter idiocy.

# Don't Count Calories

I can't tell you how many people I've surprised by telling them a food calorie (which is actually a kilocalorie, or kcal for short) is in fact a unit used to measure heat and has pretty much no relevance whatsoever to our diets. The definition of a kilocalorie is actually 'the energy needed to raise the temperature of one litre of water through one degree Celsius'. So that means your average bag of Walkers crisps contains nearly enough energy to get 2 litres of room temperature water to boiling point. Confused? I'm not surprised. Calories *are* confusing and we shouldn't be getting hung up on them. *Calor* is the Latin word for heat, and the French scientist blokey chap who invented the calorie meant it to be used as a unit of heat measurement, not something for every woman the world over to bash herself over the head with on a daily basis.

Using calories to measure nutrition is about as useful as using a ruler to check your bra size. I haven't counted a single calorie since the start of 2012 and I don't ever intend to count one again. I'm campaigning for the food industry to ditch calories all together. They honestly aren't worth the paper they're printed on.

When the calorific values of food were worked out over a century ago by an agricultural chemist called Wilbur Olin Atwater, he literally burned samples of food, and then measured the amount of energy released by the heat they produced. He worked out that protein and carbohydrate yield 4 calories per gram and fats 9 calories per gram.

But Atwater's figures don't take into account that high-protein foods such as chicken are estimated to take between ten and twenty times as much energy to digest as fats, while many highly processed or sugary foods like honey seem to barely tax the digestive system at all, meaning no extra calories are needed to digest them. High-fibre and raw unprocessed food require more chewing and are more difficult to digest, so you use up more calories eating them. In fact, up to 25 per cent of the calories in nuts like almonds may not be absorbed at all, but this is never accounted for on food labels.

If that isn't enough to convince you, consider the fact that food labels in the UK are allowed by law to be inaccurate by as much as 20 per cent. That means – playing devil's advocate and counting calories for a minute – that every day you could be consuming a fifth more calories than you intend to. Over the course of a year, that means you could be chowing down on nearly 132,000 extra calories unintentionally, or 270 Big Macs. As if calories weren't useless enough, you can't even trust them to be accurate.

The food industry has a job to do just like anyone else, but the lifestyles they sell us and the images they promote and attach to certain foods shouldn't be taken at face value. Call me a cynic, but there's a lot of lobbying that goes on in food politics. And while it may be good for the government's coffers for industry and food policy makers to be in cahoots, it sure isn't helping the health or waistlines of the nation. Take the government's 'eatwell plate': the state still reckons we should all be eating piles of starchy carbohydrates every day. The latest research indicates that this is not a very good idea at all for keeping down rates of obesity, diabetes and heart disease; but still, despite overwhelming evidence to the contrary, the government is still sticking to its eatwell plate, which appears on pretty much every hospital wall and school canteen in the UK.

I'm not usually one for conspiracy theories, but I reckon that one very big fat reason for this is that the government doesn't want to get on the wrong side of the big food companies. In America, one top professor (Walter Willett of the very prestigious School of Public Health at Harvard University) recently stated: 'Federal dietary guidelines recommending that Americans of all ages consume three cups per day of reduced fat milk or other dairy products may be influenced more by lobbying from the dairy industry than by scientific evidence.' That's not some Bristolian blonde saying it, but a professor from Harvard. If you were a cereal manufacturer, for example, wouldn't you sure as hell use whatever influence you could to keep the nation tucking into a bowl of cereal in the morning?

Even the confectionery and soft-drink producers have nothing to complain about: the NHS eatwell plate shows an 8 per cent segment containing Battenberg cake, choccies and cans of cola, making it seem as though it's okay to eat these things every single day. Put like that, it seems like utter insanity.

In short, I don't set too much store by the eatwell plate or any other government food advice, given it's always a compromise to try to keep big taxpaying food corporations on board.

If you want to have a really healthy diet, you need to know more about food. And that knowledge shouldn't just extend to meals – you need to know about ingredients. How many of us actually look at what we're buying and read the list of ingredients? Yes, we all know E numbers are nobody's friend, but you need to know what's in your food and the processes it goes through. Who knew that the pasteurization of milk, cheese and yogurt kills almost all the enzymes we need to digest it? As a rule of thumb, I use the 'If you can't spell it or pronounce it, don't eat it' mantra. So if the label says a product contains additives like sulphites, bisulphates, polyphosphates, mono-, di- and triglycerides . . . you get my gist. If it doesn't sound like plain English, it's probably not good for you and you should probably stay away from it.

Once I'd found the motivation to diet, I read everything I could get my hands on about every diet I'd ever heard of. Slowly but surely I re-educated myself to such an extent that the thought of continuing to eat like I had been eating for the last twenty-five years repulsed me.

This time, I went into losing weight with my eyes wide open. I watched documentaries on YouTube, listened to conferences with doctors from all over the world, read articles and books, watched DVDs, took courses in nutrition – the whole nine yards. You could say I was trying to delay the inevitable bit where I had to get off my bum and move, and maybe that was part of it. But I researched weight, diets, exercise and metabolism like I was going on *The $64,000 Question*. Start by watching some of Dr Robert Lustig's talks on YouTube: you'll be surprised at what you'll learn in just a few minutes.

I thought long and hard about what I wanted to eat and how I wanted to eat. I spent hours investigating which kind of exercise I wanted to do. Through my research I found a diet that made sense to me – and I don't mean the calorie-counting, faddy diets you've probably tried already. I mean a new way of eating that is healthy and natural, that looks after your body and gives you energy. It will help you lose weight, but it makes nutritional sense on so many other levels as well.

In this step I'm going to explain the principles of the diet. One of the most powerful weapons in your weight-loss journey will be knowledge. There's no substitute for it. You need to know why you've chosen to eat what you have, why it will work and how it will work. Knowledge will stop you making the wrong decisions in the supermarket or at a restaurant. I know I chose what was right for me. How? Look at me – it worked.

I'm also going to give you meal plans and recipes and share my own experiences to help you through the first few weeks. I'll give tips on dealing with cravings if you get them and show you how to stay motivated. You don't have to go hungry, you don't have to count calories. And, best of all, you get one day a week to eat anything you like.

# SIX

# Why the Diet Works

As I did my research into diets, I found that the ones making the most sense were based on the idea of going back to our Stone Age roots and eating food our bodies were adapted for. Back then we ate plenty of protein, but minimal grain-based and processed carbs, like white bread and white rice for instance, which just weren't around. I learned that I'd been poisoning myself for years with all the processed rubbish I ate, denying my body the nutrition it needed. So I worked out a plan that suited me and now I live by the motto: if you can't pick it or kill it, don't eat it. I eat entirely natural foods that haven't been processed – they haven't been refined or pasteurized or prepared. The protein, carbohydrates and sugars I eat are all as close to their natural state as they can be when I eat them. I eat plenty of raw veggies and salads. The only process I put my food through is to cook it. In short, I eat like we would have done thousands of years ago, when kebab shops and McDonald's didn't exist, and we only had fire to cook with.

# Protein – Why We Need to Eat More

Only 15 per cent of energy in the average modern diet comes from protein, but thousands of years ago it was more like 35 per cent. When was the last time you opened a textbook and saw a fat caveman or woman? Just look at Raquel Welch and her *One Million Years B.C.* bod.

Protein was overlooked as an important nutrient for years while we all obsessed about eating too many calories or too much fat. For ages everyone went down the wrong road with diets that were high in carbs. But now scientists are realizing that protein is a key nutrient for health, and we need to be sure we get enough in our daily diet, especially when we're trying to lose weight as it's vital for making and maintaining the lean muscle tissue that keeps our metabolic rate higher. More than that, it is the golden bullet in hunger management; it's far better at keeping you filled up than either carbohydrates or fat. The diet I follow includes plenty of protein.

# Carbs – Why We Need to Eat Less

Carbohydrates are found in lots of foods from vegetables, with the highest quantities found in root vegetables such as potatoes (and therefore crisps), to grains like rice and wheat (including pasta, bread and biscuits), and even bananas. Carbohydrates give us energy but if you eat more than you can burn off – which is what we do in the West – then your body stores the excess as fat. Excess carbs are more likely to end up making a beeline for your belly area than excess fats or protein. So while foods high in carbohydrates *can* be an integral part of a healthy diet, they've been given way too much prominence in the past and research shows that eating too many of the wrong sorts of carbohydrate not only contributes to weight gain and interferes with weight loss but also promotes diabetes and heart disease.

If you pile your plate with the refined sort – white rice, cotton-woolly white bread or those puffed corn or maize savoury snacks, for instance – you're eating almost pure starch, and as far as your body is concerned you might as well be eating spoonfuls of white sugar straight from the packet.

That's because they are processed and, bereft of the high-fibre bran layer and vitamin-rich germ, grains provide mostly fast-releasing energy and not much else. So you'll get a quick rush of glucose into your blood stream, perking you up for a while, but later you'll feel famished and jittery, looking for your next food fix. Even worse, these fast-releasing grains trigger large releases of insulin, and this in turn is linked with the laying down of dangerous hormonally-active fat that not only means you can't do up the waist on your jeans but puts you at a higher risk of diabetes, high blood pressure, heart disease and strokes. In short, while some grains can be really good for you, the wrong sort can mean your waistline won't shrink and may even get bigger. My diet cuts out all processed carbs and that is probably one of the biggest adjustments you will have to make – so many of us live on cereal and toast for breakfast, sandwiches for lunch and pasta or pizza for dinner. I promise you'll soon get used to it.

Whole grain carbs – the type found in wholemeal bread, brown rice and wholewheat pasta – do deliver vitamins, minerals, fibre and a host of other important nutrients, but there are some experts and scientists who maintain our bodies just haven't evolved fast enough to deal with grains at all, even whole grains. They argue that we never grew them for consumption when we all wore loincloths, so our bodies can't metabolize them properly now. But I've come round to thinking that it is OK to have the whole grains in modest quantities. Growing crops is what enabled settlements of people to gather in one place and civilizations to develop, and I for one am glad that bread was invented and we're not all still running around in animal skins scavenging a few berries and clubbing woolly mammoths.

Interestingly, in 1991 when they opened up Ötzi, that ice man they found in the Alps who lived over 5,000 years ago, they found evidence of a grain meal inside him, so I don't think we can all go around claiming we're 'far too prehistoric, darling' to indulge in a bit of wheat. It's possible that, for some of us, our bodies deal with grains better than others, and this is something you can find out by keeping a food diary and seeing how grain intake affects your waistline, energy levels and weight.

I believe that unprocessed whole grains are an important part of my diet, adding variety and interest to meals, keeping me on an even keel energy-wise, keeping my bowel movements regular and providing essential nutrients. So while I'll go out of my way to avoid the refined ones, I'm happy keeping unprocessed whole grain types in my way of eating, like old-fashioned milled oats (not the instant sort), quinoa (technically a seed, but let's not split hairs here), and a smidge of brown rice. My top tip would be to combine healthy grain foods with a source of protein to keep hunger at bay and energy levels steadier. So if you're eating a slice of rye bread for breakfast, have some scrambled eggs and smoked salmon or lean ham with it.

I eat whole grains maybe once or twice a week – you could have them more often if they suit you, but I've found too much gluten doesn't agree with me. I introduced them gradually to my diet and made sure I noted down in my food diary what they did for my energy levels, waistline and skin. Do the same and you'll learn which ones work for you and which ones you should steer clear of.

So what is gluten? It's a protein composite found in wheat, rye and barley. Sounds easy to avoid doesn't it? But that means most bread, pasta, breakfast cereals, flour, pizza, cakes and biscuits. Around one in a hundred people in the UK have coeliac disease which is a proper full-blown adverse reaction to the gluten in these foods. If you're a coeliac, the body mistakes the substances inside gluten as a threat and attacks them. This damages the surface of the small intestines, disrupting your ability to absorb the nutrients from food your body needs.

That's pretty nasty stuff, and if you are diagnosed with coeliac disease you need to avoid every scrap of gluten in your diet or risk becoming really ill. But what if you're not a coeliac, but still find that eating too much bread, pasta or cereal makes you feel bleugh? If that's you, then there's a possibility that you have non-coeliac gluten sensitivity like me. This has been proposed as a separate condition from coeliac disease – not as bad, and not causing any permanent damage to your gut, but still making you feel bloated, uncomfortable and generally a bit out of sorts when you eat more gluten than you can personally tolerate. Those who work in the field of gluten sensitivity suggest anywhere between 7 and 30 per cent of us may have it. What's more, a third of those affected report brain fog and fatigue as symptoms, so it can mess with your head as well as your gut.

I for one find that eating too much gluten makes me feel gross both physically and mentally, so I'd advise you if you're eating lots – and those wheat-based foods really accumulate – you cut down and try gluten-free alternatives instead. There's a gluten-free aisle in every supermarket which I bet you just rush by, but take a wander down there and, I promise you, you'll be pleasantly surprised.

Root vegetables (including sweet potatoes, turnips, beetroot, onions and celeriac) contain the healthier carbs and fibre which make them slower to digest and keep you fuller for longer. These are fab and my diet is packed with them. The exception to the rule is the not-so-humble potato. They contain masses of starchy carbohydrates which are quickly released. Mashed spuds, for example, can raise your blood sugar as quickly as sugar can. Sweet potatoes are OK though and you can get away with small amounts of boiled new potatoes with their skins on too.

I don't keep any bad carbs in the house, but I do keep tons of root veg and some bananas. That way, when I'm craving carbs, there's no option but for me to reach for the good ones.

The bottom line is that any carbs that aren't in the form of whole vegetables or fruit should be treated with caution and avoided if you're trying to lose weight. And in order to lose weight and stay slim you should only have one fist-sized portion of high carb foods like grains and sweet potatoes a day.

# Sugar

It turns out that sugar is hidden away absolutely everywhere in food products, and it can cause way more problems than just extra visits to the dentist. Some obesity experts, like Professor Robert

Lustig from the University of California at San Francisco, who I mentioned earlier, have even labelled sugar a toxin.

The UK chocolate confectionery industry is worth £4,000 billion a year, and that's just chocolate. Sugar's in literally everything. Think your brown bread is healthy? There's 1.6 grams of sugar in every slice. Ever thought your bagel tasted a bit sweet? That's because a plain one can have the equivalent of a whole sugar cube (4.8 grams) inside it. Reckon baked beans represent one of your five a day? They may well do, but they'll also deliver you a 9.9-gram hit of sugar per portion. Think you're safe with butter? There could still be small traces of sugar in it from the high fructose levels in some cattle feed. We all know a strawberry milkshake from McDonald's is going to contain sugar, right? But what if I told you a large one has sixteen cubes of sugar in it?

The white stuff contributes to over 35 million deaths every year, costs the NHS over £4 billion a year and can lead to a host of health conditions, including type 2 diabetes, heart disease, strokes, liver problems and even certain types of cancer. Unless we tackle the UK's sugar addiction, there's a real risk we could bankrupt our health service. There's emerging evidence to suggest that high-sugar diets may promote some cancers: the theory goes that glucose, which makes up around 50 per cent of the sucrose and high-fructose corn syrup used to sweeten foods, creates repeated spikes of insulin, which in turn give tumours with insulin receptors – those of the breast and colon, for example – a greater chance to hijack the flow of glucose in the blood stream and use it to grow.

Sugar suppresses the immune system, so in addition to being the cause of plenty of physical conditions and illnesses, it also leaves our systems open to attack from many other health problems. When we imbibe the white stuff, neurotransmitters in the brain react the same way as they do when we drink alcohol or take drugs. Over the years we become tolerant to it and need to increase consumption to get same the hit off it as we once did. Put simply: Sugar. Can. Kill. You. Slowly.

As if all that weren't bad enough, sugar also ages you and kills off the elasticity in your skin, so in addition to making you ill, it makes you look old. I honestly think that the reason I haven't been left with rolls of loose skin is because I gave up the white stuff before I'd even started losing weight. It was one of the first things I did and so the elasticity returned to my skin.

I knew I loved sugar, and had done since I was a child, but when I looked into exactly how much I consumed, I was shocked. Look at the labels on your food: it's in everything. Ever bought one of those huge tubs of 'low fat' yogurt? They're crammed with over 20 per cent of our recommended daily intake of sugar. Sugar is one of the biggest killers in the UK, but we laugh and joke about it in a way we don't about alcohol and drug addiction. People use sugar addiction as a punchline, but the joke is on us.

On my one-day-a-week treat days, I will normally have a few glasses of bubbly or some other sweet treat, but otherwise my diet is totally sugar free, other than naturally occurring fructose in whole fruit – and has been for nearly two years. I still crave it and I always will, but my habits have now changed. I spent over twenty years as a sugar addict, and I'll always be in recovery because it's impossible to cure yourself of an addiction. I still can't have it in the house because I know the temptation is too much. You may think I've just got a sweet tooth, and that because you like crackers and cheese or crisps more than you like choccie buttons, you're not an addict. But there's sugar in most crackers (except for oatcakes), in cheeses, even in crisps. And if you're going to succeed in shifting the extra pounds that have plagued you for years, you need to know how much of the white stuff you're eating and how responsible it is for you getting to the point you're at.

Look at your food labels and use your food diary: write down everything you eat which contains sugar and try to work out the percentage of your recommended daily amount you're eating. I promise the results will shock and surprise you. To be healthy, 'added' sugars, those used to add extra sweetness to food, or in honeys, syrups and fruit juices, shouldn't make up more than 10 per cent of the energy we get from food – that's 50 grams, or 10 cubes a day. Just one 500ml bottle of cola will get you to this limit. And before you think 'I know all of that', consider that you'll be halfway to your daily maximum by the time you've breakfasted on a bowl of bran flakes and a glass of orange juice, which may have been your go-to healthy breakfast in the past. Even freshly-squeezed fruit juice, with nothing added, should be avoided. Without the fibre, the fructose in the fruit is metabolized more quickly. Plus the chances are that a glassful of juice contains several fruit, more than you would eat if whole, thereby upping your fructose intake.

The sugars in milk, vegetables and whole (non-juiced) fruits are much more innocuous, so if you're getting much of your sugar from these sources, you can eat up to 18 cubes or 90 grams daily (the guideline daily amount or GDA for total sugars) safely. Basically, if you cut out processed sugar and have one portion of fruit a day, plus small amounts of milk in tea or coffee, you don't need to worry about exceeding this limit. I promise you that once you cut processed sugars out of your diet, an apple will taste out of this world.

## ARE YOU AT WAR WITH THE WHITE STUFF?

If you answer yes to three or more of these statements, you'll benefit from ditching sugar from your diet.

1. Have you ever gone out late at night, travelled a considerable distance or overcome obstacles in your quest for sugar?
2. Does eating sweet treats make you happy even after a bad day?
3. Is a sweet treat planned every day as part of your diet?
4. Have you ever tried to limit the amount of sugar you eat?
5. Do you lie or hide the amount of sugar you scoff?
6. Would your friends and family describe your palate as sweet?
7. Can you leave biscuits in the barrel or sweets in the jar, or do you have to eat the lot?
8. On previous diets have you refused or found it hard to lower your sugar intake?
9. Do you find it hard to turn down dessert at a restaurant?

Sugar fuels every single cell in our brains. In studies looking into addiction and how it affects us, rats that binged on sugar were shown to have experienced brain changes similar to drug withdrawal. In humans, pictures of milkshakes alone triggered brain effects like those seen in drug addicts. It was strongest in female subjects, whose answers showed they were more hooked on eating. Do you need any more incentive to look at how the sugar you're eating is affecting your waistline and your brain too?

If this seems too hard, you can use stevia or xylitol as alternatives to sugar so you can still enjoy your cup of tea, plus there are tips on how to handle any cravings in Chapter 9 (see page 191).

# Dairy

It's not rocket science to point out that sugar is bad for you. But what if I told you that dairy might not be much better? We're the only species on the planet that drinks milk past infancy and definitely the only ones who drink the milk of a totally different species. In spite of the fact that we're told that dairy foods contain the calcium we need for strong bones, in the UK we have higher rates of osteoporosis than nations that never touch dairy, and we are certainly not any healthier all round. Looking at it like this, those ads and government schemes that try to get us drinking gallons of milk look more like propaganda from the dairy industry than a genuine attempt to improve our health. Makes you think twice about your bowl of Rice Krispies in the morning, doesn't it?

I had suffered with bloating all my life; even when I ditched sugar, I still had bloating and stomach cramps. Enter Google again, stage left. After searching long and hard on the internet, I realized my symptoms fit with the theory that I might be slightly lactose intolerant – basically I don't have as much as everyone else of the right enzyme (called lactase) in my gut to break down the sugar (called lactose) found in all dairy products, from milk and cheese to yogurt and, yep, Ben & Jerry's.

Having proved to myself I could ditch the other white stuff, I wondered how hard it would be to come off dairy for a week or two and see if it made a difference. There are tons of milk substitutes out there, from almond milk to rice milk, so no one ever need sacrifice their morning cuppa – that would be above and beyond the call of duty. Just sneak a quick peek at the pack to make sure your chosen substitute is calcium-fortified and you're good to go dairy free. I've always loved ice-cream, but I'm as happy with a mango sorbet as with a bowl of Neapolitan, so it didn't seem too much of a stretch. Besides, when you start changing your diet for the better and see and feel the difference, you're inspired to keep going and see what else you can fix and where else you may have been going wrong all these years.

Within 72 hours of giving up all dairy, the change was incredible. I used to wake up every day with a blocked nose, and would always feel crampy and achy until a trip to the toilet first thing in the morning. Those symptoms were gone. Not only that, but within a few days of ditching dairy I noticed my waist literally shrinking as the gassy bloating disappeared.

You see, we're conditioned to think of processed food as being brightly packaged stuff in supermarkets and petrol stations that's easy to identify. We know it's bad for us and most of us reckon we could spot it a mile off. But milk and cheese are some of the most processed foods in your supermarket aisles. They both go through a pasteurization process, and that destroys lots of the essential proteins, vitamins and enzymes that assist digestion. Getting rid of them makes it that bit harder for our systems to digest these foods and puts more of a strain on the delicate balance in our systems.

After my fortnight off dairy, I felt like a new woman. The spots I'd been battling for weeks had gone, my skin was glowing, my stomach was smaller, I was sleeping better, the old bowel movements were more regular, I had more energy – and I'd developed a real penchant for almond-milk porridge. Now I get my calcium from eating leafy greens like cabbage and broccoli, and my vitamin D (which helps us absorb it) from fish and eggs.

But no sooner had I detoxed from dairy than I decided to do an experiment to see if my self-diagnosis of mild lactose intolerance was correct. I thought I'd be OK performing said experiment on the train up to London for a meeting. The buffet car didn't have any almond milk and I was gagging for a coffee. I was pretty sure I was intolerant, but then I'd been drinking milk and eating cheese, yogurt and ice-cream for twenty-five years and had only been off it a couple of weeks – what harm could a drop of milk in the top of my filter coffee do?

Quite a lot, it turns out. I spent the journey from Bath Spa to London Paddington in the toilet of the 11.13 First Great Western train with the worst stomach cramps I've ever had. If you decide to ditch dairy and then reintroduce it, don't make the same mistake I did; wait until you're in the safety of your own home in close proximity to your bathroom. I'd also advise anyone to ditch dairy for a while see if it makes a difference to your diet. If you suffer from any of the following symptoms, lactose intolerance may be the root cause:

- bloating
- gas
- diarrhoea
- nasal congestion
- stomach cramps
- fatigue
- acne
- hives
- restless sleep
- respiratory disorders, shortness of breath
- hay fever

My experiment reinforced my belief that I've got lactose-intolerant tendencies (you can also be intolerant or allergic to the proteins in milk, but bloating, diarrhoea and cramps usually indicate it's the lactose sugar you have a problem with). And when you have lactose intolerance, you've got a choice – you either keep putting up with the discomfort and eating little bits of dairy to try to keep whatever small amount of lactose-digesting capacity you have left still working, or ditch it all together and say goodbye to the bloated tum. I still have dairy very occasionally, but 98 per cent of my diet is dairy free. I'm much healthier for it and I'd recommend you do the same. I certainly feel a million times better for it.

I ditched dairy for three months before introducing it back very slowly. If you take dairy out of your diet completely, be careful about when and where you decide to reintroduce it. Your ability to digest lactose will dwindle from not much to not at all, meaning that if you accidentally eat some dairy you could discover it in the unpleasant and embarrassing way that I found out on my train trip. But embrace the no-dairy way completely for the first few months of your new eating plan, and your stomach and waistline will thank you for it always.

# Alcohol

One of the hardest parts of this journey was changing my relationship with alcohol. It won't come as a surprise that I haven't been a saint all my life when it comes to booze. I spent almost every weekend from my late teens to my mid-twenties getting well and truly mullered. I'd wake up after benders filled with self-loathing, dreading someone telling me exactly how I'd made a fool of myself the previous night. I'd stuff my face with rubbish throughout the day before doing it all again the next night. Looking back, I can see I was drinking like a fish to give me confidence. When I could barely see straight, I couldn't feel people looking at the fat girl I was. But all that my boozing did was rob me of the motivation to do anything about my weight. And to add insult to injury, it made me even fatter because it is high in sugar. When I ditched the booze, I lost mates. It's not nice to admit it but some of them didn't care for the new Josie. They weren't interested in my suggestions of a trip to the cinema in place of some Jägerbombs. It hurt at the time but with hindsight I can see they weren't proper mates and I'm glad they're not in my life anymore.

Don't get me wrong, I still like the odd tipple only now, instead of eight cheeky ciders and some shots every weekend, I treat myself to a nice bottle of champagne once or twice a month. I'm spending way less on booze than I used to and because champagne is fermented differently, it doesn't contain as much sugar as your regular vino. And if I overindulge on a treat day, I juice the next – picking anything from my veg drawer, perhaps adding one piece of fruit. It cures my hangover within a few gulps. If you're a big boozer like I was, use the money you would spend on Cheeky Vimtos to buy a juicer – you'll thank me for it in the long run.

If you can't afford champagne, a couple of small glasses of wine on your treat day won't hurt. I'm sure you know that the recommended amount of alcohol for a woman per week is 14 units, and 21 for men – now that doesn't mean you can have it all in one go if you've been off the booze the rest of the week! The recommended intake per day for a woman is no more than 2–3 units (that's roughly one 175ml glass of wine) or 3–4 units for men (that's a pint and a half of 4 per cent beer). Doctors say you should have two days a week without any alcohol anyway and you should definitely limit your intake if you want to lose weight. I recommend keeping it for your treat day only.

# Don't be Scared

By now you might be panicking that if you can't have cornflakes and toast for breakfast or a sandwich for lunch, you won't be able to eat anything. Don't worry! In the next chapter I'm going to show you all the lovely food you *can* eat, as well as what you can't. And in addition to the recipes I've provided in this book, there will be lots of others on my new website www.slimmables.com which will be up and running in spring 2013.

When I was working out my healthy eating plan, I spent hours if not days poring over every food website I could find. I tried Gwyneth Paltrow's recipes, but her perfect body, stunning hair and gorgeous bloke and family made me feel a bit crap. So instead of reading what other people did and how others cooked their way slinky, I got off my shrinking backside and popped down my local high street. I bought and tried different fruits and vegetables every week.

I'd research a vegetable I knew I wanted to try, like the humble sweet potato, and would buy loads of them. I'd try them every which way: cooked with some chicken in a pan and some mushrooms; sliced and dusted in ground cumin then roasted. Or with some mackerel or a piece of cod for fish and chips Josie-style, or sliced and piled into a dish cooked with some stock and poached chicken. I experimented. Not everything was a resounding success – my avocado porridge won't be hitting the high street any time soon – but I took my time, learned about foods, cooking processes and ingredients and tried different things.

Before I became the domestic goddess I am now, I started off with trays of root veg bought ready to cook from the supermarket with a piece of salmon on top. But I soon grew in confidence and started making salads with poached eggs and asparagus or pancakes with bananas and nuts. I'm no Gwyneth (don't let the blonde hair fool you), but I know cooking well comes from experimenting and building up your confidence. In Chapter 8 there are some of my favourite recipes, the tried and tested ones I know and love.

If you've been living off processed food, you may not have tried or even heard of some of the fruits and vegetables you can eat; but if you're going to love food in a healthier way, you need to expand your palate and investigate new flavours, new tastes, new textures and new ingredients. On average people lose half their taste receptors by the time they turn twenty, so your palate may already be pretty dulled; introducing it to new flavours and tastes will help keep you motivated.

Some of the ingredients may not be up your street, but don't let that put you off. It's all about substituting. Don't like prawns? Switch them for chicken breast. Don't fancy butternut squash? Swap it for sweet potato or pumpkin. Find your own rhythm and you're far more likely to stick to an eating plan than if I, or anyone else, tell you what you must and must not cook, what you can and cannot avoid. Only by learning about foods and their properties, and how they'll help your body, can you start figuring out how to put recipes together for yourself that will work for you and your body.

It's said that kids need to try something on average ten times before they accept the new flavour on their palate and form a taste for it. There's no evidence it's any different for us adults, so persevere with new flavours and tastes. Besides, if you're denying yourself your usual fix of biscuits, crisps or ice-cream, you need to make sure your taste buds are kept stimulated by using different textures, flavours and colours.

Sometimes I have hours and days off in a row when I have time to stock up the fridge and freezer with marinades and dressings I know will last, or breakfast granola bars I can grab when I get busy. Sometimes breakfast has to be a banana and a handful of nuts because it's all I've got time for. Sometimes dinner has to be a bagged salad with some prawns chucked in and a jacket sweet potato. But if you've got a good few dressings stocked in the fridge, you can transform even the most humble combination of seafood and leaves into something amazing.

Think about textures, too. Your porridge will be so much more interesting with a few ground nuts sprinkled on top. Soup seems so much more exciting with a bit of creamy coconut milk swirled on top at the last moment. We eat with our eyes and our taste buds, but our mouths are as excited by textures as our eyes are by the colour of food. We like a bit of texture and difference, so when your dinner is ready, ask yourself if it might benefit from something sprinkled or flaked on top.

My diet now, apart from my treat days, contains lots of lean protein with plenty of veggies, no processed junk, very little dairy, a small amount of grains and no added sugar. I reckon that definitely qualifies me to wear Raquel's animal-print bikini! I promise I didn't choose it just because it looked like the sort of diet my thinspiration cavewoman would be on; but the more I've developed my plan to suit myself, the more I've realized restrictive diets that are prescriptive down to the letter are the ones we're destined to fail at. Every diet, even this one, needs to be approached with knowledge and foresight. Take elements that suit you and adapt ones that don't. I spent months re-educating my brain in order to change my body. The way I eat now has tons of benefits but no set rules, which for me is the best way to diet. Nothing feels off limits, nothing feels 'naughty' and I know far more about what I've eaten in the last two years than I did in the previous twenty-seven combined.

If you'd told the old me I wasn't allowed to have something, I'd instantly start craving it. Now, eating what I like, when I like, as long as it's natural and not processed, means my diet is easy even for food-obsessed me to stick to. I promise you hand on heart, if you give it a go you can reap the same health and weight-loss benefits as I have.

The way I eat now and the food choices I make leave me with so many options: I don't restrict myself, I just simply find the healthy alternative to foods I crave. If I find myself wanting a Mars bar, I reach for the homemade almond blondies on page 176. If I walk past the chip shop and feel hungry, I cook myself some sweet-potato fries with cumin and some homemade salsa. I don't get the mood swings that used to plague me, I have energy levels I haven't had since I was a kid and I never, ever go hungry.

Keeping my body and brain working together as one makes me feel strong and healthy, and I've been on my diet for so long that going back to the old way I ate makes me feel queasy just thinking about it. I don't want to pollute my body with the food I once ate. I am no longer a slave to food. I love food and I embrace food and I still eat boatloads of it, but I eat the right clean healthy-living foods and I work out.

If you only take one thing away from these pages, though, let it be that cutting down on processed crap and switching to fresh wholesome food, including lots of appetite-curbing protein, can make a world of difference to your weight and health. I'm living proof of that.

# Cold Turkey v. Gradual Changes

Before we get on to the diet itself, which is going to involve giving up sugar, you might want to consider whether it is too hard for you to go cold turkey. Honestly? I'd love everyone in the world to ditch sugar from their diet right now. I have no sympathy for all those poor dentists who would go out of business. But the reality is that doing what I did and going cold turkey is hard. Very hard. It's not impossible – if I can do it, anyone can – but you've got to really want it and devote yourself to it until you're in control of your cravings rather than the other way round.

There's more than one way to skin a sweet potato, though. If it seems too much of an ask to change things forever right now, you can still make changes – just do it gradually over a matter of weeks or months rather than hours and days. Cutting down slowly will be gentler on your system and may assuage some of the more serious side effects I had to contend with. I've persuaded lots of my mates to go cold turkey, and while they've thanked me for it in the long run, there are other friends who've preferred to take things slowly.

You're training your body; why not train your mind too? I'm proof we don't need sugar as much as we may think we do. If you can retrain your body to enjoy and even look forward to exercise, then apply the same mentality to your taste buds. Train them to enjoy things that aren't as sweet. It takes twenty-one days for us to form a habit. If you don't believe me, try this experiment: when you brush your teeth every morning and evening, start doing it on the opposite side first. If you brush to the right first, start brushing to the left, and vice versa. You'll have to remind yourself for what seems like ages to do it, but I guarantee you, if you do it for twenty-one days, by day twenty-two you'll have totally changed the way you brush your teeth. Just three weeks is long enough for you to change your habits forever.

You're trying to change your lifelong associations with food and cravings you've had for a decade or more. If going cold turkey feels a bit too daunting, take it slowly and try cutting out one sweet food from your diet each week. Start off slowly by reducing the amount of sugar in your coffee or cereal, or turn down the offer of a pudding menu when you're out for dinner, or limit yourself to one or two bars of chocolate a week instead of two a day. Over time, you will lose your need for that sugar taste and your body and brain will adapt to live without it. It'll seem like a daunting task to begin with, but in a few weeks you'll be surprised at how fast you've adapted and how little your body needs the sweet stuff. In the grand old scheme of things, twenty-one days is nothing, but your body, your waistline and your doctor will thank you for it for the rest of your life.

I'm an all-or-nothing kind of girl, though, so other than on my treat days, I banned processed sugar from my diet right from day one. I'd tried cutting down before and knew it didn't work for me; that's not to say it won't work for you. Giving myself a treat day made my diet easier to stick to. It took about three weeks for my taste buds to start changing. Once my palate was cleansed of added sugar, I started to taste naturally occurring sugars more. The once bland apple I'd forced down at lunchtime in an attempt to be healthy now seemed packed with flavour and different varieties were a treat to taste. I used to crave a chocolate hit; now I crave granola, fruit and lots of natural yogurt. It took a while, but my taste buds eventually woke up after years of being stifled by artificial flavours and overwhelming sweetness.

Let protein lend a hand too. You'll be more susceptible to giving in to cravings when you're hungry. Foods high in protein will leave you feeling fuller for longer, so the temptation to eat sugar won't come as often and may be easier to deal with when it does descend. I shocked my system when I lost weight because I knew I had to go hard or go home. I'd tried the softly, gently approach before, but it had never worked for me and whatever weight I lost had always found its way back to my bum, tum and thighs. But you don't have to approach losing weight with an all-or-nothing mentality. I did what suited me. It may suit you too; but if it doesn't, don't be scared to find your own route to eating better and being healthier.

Making gradual changes will be easier on your system and help you phase out bad habits and foods over time, which will make your diet easier to stick to longer term. If you're a full-English-in-the-morning bird, me telling you to ditch it for porridge isn't going to work, is it? Like any mare I've ever ridden, I need to break you in gently.

If you love a big breakfast, ditch the toast to start off with. Then start grilling your bacon rather than frying it. You probably won't notice a scrap of difference, but you'll be making a healthier choice right away. Once you're used to that, start to poach your eggs instead of frying them; they're more delicious this way anyway, and you'll also be avoiding the oil or butter you fry them in. Or if you must fry them, use a brush of coconut oil in a good non-stick pan rather than vegetable oil. When you're used to your new-style bacon and eggs, start to grill your tomatoes and mushrooms rather than frying them. Neither needs the excess oil you fry them in, and they stand a better chance of keeping more of their natural nutrients this way. Then, after a few weeks, add a piece of fruit when you're finished. Hey presto! In a matter of weeks, you've switched your entire full English breakfast for something far healthier, and it won't have felt too much like a wrench because you'll have done it gradually. Don't be scared to find your own way: you're not just dieting, you're educating yourself forever. You need to experiment to find the right fit for you, because there'll be no going back.

I used to separate all my food choices into four categories; unhealthy, average, healthy and bloody healthy. My aim was to get from 'unhealthy', which I was constantly stuck in, to 'bloody healthy', which is where I hang out most of the time now.

Take lunch. If you're a Big Mac and fries type for lunch or dinner, switch to a homemade chicken-breast burger with homemade chips for your 'average' choice, then to chicken breast with sweet-potato fries with cumin for the 'healthy' version, then to a steamed chicken breast with steamed veggies for the 'bloody healthy' version.

If you take baby steps and make little changes, you're far more likely to stick to your diet than if you make broad sweeping changes that could leave you with cravings so bad you'd kill your granny for a Malted Milk biscuit. I know I don't need to tell you that, but maybe you need to be reminded. It's not easy losing weight. There's a lot to think about, take in, learn and consider. You're trying to change habits you didn't even know you had and find new ways to think about food after a lifetime of seeing it the same way. Don't crucify yourself trying to fix your diet overnight: the likelihood is that you'll make bad choices, end up with a totally boring and uninspiring new 'healthy' diet and ditch the whole idea before you've even lost a few pounds.

So, if you're a fan of spaghetti bolognese with parmesan, switch to wholewheat spaghetti with quality beef mince and parmesan, then ditch the parmesan, then switch to making your 'spaghetti' out of a courgette, thinly sliced and then the slices cut into long strips.

If you love a portion of chips, switch them for potato wedges with rapeseed oil, then sweet-potato chips, then baked sweet-potato wedges and some salsa.

Going cold turkey was tough, but I knew I had to do it in order to make it. If this is your first shot at losing weight and you know you can do it gradually, be my guest. It wasn't my first time and I knew doing it gradually didn't work for me. Like I said, we're all different and it's about finding what's right and what works for you. Having said that, if you take the gradual approach, the weight won't come off as quickly – if that is going to affect your motivation, then you are better off going cold turkey like I did.

# SEVEN

# Starting the Diet – What to Eat and Meal Plans

## The Rules

All you have to do is eat the foods you are allowed for six days a week, and then you can eat what you like on your treat day. If you prefer, you could swap a day off the diet for an individual breakfast, lunch and dinner off at different times during the week. Every Sunday I make a massive roast with all the trimmings and enjoy it with Lukey and the family. I make roast potatoes with butter and goose fat or dripping, honey roast my root vegetables, butter my freshly picked veg, gorge myself on crackling or crispy chicken skin and round it all off with a nice pud, usually served with some double cream or custard. And I don't feel one iota of guilt. If I could get away with it, I'd lick the plate at the end of it. Treat days mean I don't find it hard to stick to eating right the other six days of the week. No matter how dejected I get, I'm always able to remind myself I'm at best only six days away from a treat. Thinking that way makes it easier for me to stick to being good. In fact, having a treat day on Sunday makes me want to work extra hard when I exercise on Monday.

From day one I decided I'd take twenty-four hours off each week. I honestly don't remember whether it was because I thought I couldn't sustain it for seven days a week, or whether I was scared to give it a try. It just seemed like a good way to stay motivated. It makes it easier to go cold turkey, too, when you know there's a treat day just around the corner. But, bizarrely, some Sundays I don't want to take a day off. I'll admit sometimes I go to bed on a Saturday night dreaming about the thought of a bacon butty the next morning and salivating. But sometimes I decide to ditch my day off in favour of a good workout and my normal way of eating.

Take it from someone who's tried every diet under the sun: giving yourself hard and solid rules and strict parameters will only make things really bloody hard. If you give yourself some wiggle room, it'll be easier to keep to what you're doing.

Stick to three main meals a day. Don't skip breakfast; you can eat it later in the morning if you're one of those people who just can't face food when you wake up. If you get hungry between meals, check to see if the hunger is real and not your brain playing tricks because you're stressed, bored or tired. I cover how to deal with cravings in Chapter 9. Sometimes we mistake thirst for hunger, so drink some water, wait half an hour and if you still feel the same way then have a healthy snack (see page 199 for examples). Read the early chapters again if you think you are in danger of letting your brain sabotage your regime.

You can fill your plate with vegetables from the approved list, but stick to the recommended portion size for protein: the size of a pack of cards for meat, poultry and fish. And only one portion of high carb food a day.

## THE FOODS YOU WANT TO EAT

With all the delicious ingredients I've listed below, you won't feel like you're limited at all when it comes to your food choices, and more importantly you won't feel hungry or dissatisfied. Where you can, stick to buying from markets and your local greengrocers, butchers and fishmongers – you'll be surprised at how competitive the prices are these days. Try and eat seasonally: that means no strawberries or asparagus in December. Your shopping bill will be cheaper this way and your diet will vary naturally with the seasons, meaning you're less likely to get bored of eating the same old stuff. Make sure you wash all fruit and veg before consuming or cooking.

### Meat and poultry

Always buy the best-quality meat and poultry you can – free range and organic when possible. I know everyone says that; but if you can't afford a decent bit of steak, make my lush liver recipe on page 160 instead and use your cash to get good-quality liver. Or if you've never tried it, ask your butcher for feather blade steak or flat iron – it's a tougher cut but flash fries beautifully. The better the quality of meat, the better the taste, and usually the better it's been treated. Besides, after drowning my palate in processed flavours for so long, feeding it the best quality meat I can afford is the least I can do. Avoid processed meats like cheap sausages, burgers and salami, as they're usually high in salt, sugar and preservatives; processed meats have also been linked to certain types of cancer.

Types of meat and poultry to include in your diet: any fresh, unprocessed meat and poultry. Good quality sausages and bacon in moderation.

### Fish and seafood

White fish is an excellent source of low-fat protein, and oily fish – like salmon, sardines and mackerel – is a great source of omega-3, especially if it is caught in the wild. Omega-3 is a fatty acid which is vital for a healthy metabolism and is believed to help ward off cancer and cardio-vascular disease. Farmed fish are slightly less good for you but still worth eating. Swordfish and shark should be avoided if you are concerned with mercury levels. Tinned fish like herrings and sardines can be an inexpensive way to enjoy the healthier wild type of fish, but I've learned to be a bit wary of eating lots of canned fish because cans may contain a toxin called BPA in the inner lining. It can potentially mess with your hormone levels, so if you go for 'tinned' fish, try Aldi and Lidl, who usually sell it in glass jars instead of tins.

Types of fish and shellfish to include: any kind.

### Eggs

Types of egg to include: all eggs are fine to eat.

### Fruit

Fruit is packed with nutrients and antioxidants, but you should limit intake for weight-loss as most kinds of fruit are high in the naturally occurring sugar fructose. Buy seasonally and organic if you've got the cash, but don't worry if not – just make sure you give the skin a good wash to remove any dirt, chemicals and pesticides. And don't think of fruit as just a sweet food; my pork and apricot recipe on page 165 shows you it can be used in plenty of savoury dishes too. Dried fruit is very high in sugar and should be eaten in tiny (1 tablespoon) portions only.

Types of fruit to include: any kind but just one portion (a handful if it's fresh, a tablespoon if it's dried) a day.

*Vegetables*

Nearly all vegetables are beneficial to health and contain the carbohydrates you need. They should form a large part of your diet. The exception is white potatoes, as we've seen. I love sweet potato as a substitute but it is quite high in carbs so limit your intake. And fresh peas and green beans are legumes – see pages 107–8 for guidelines. Most of the time, try to stick to vegetables with a high water content, which is most of those below, and root vegetables which are not quite so starchy.

Types of vegetables to eat:

- artichoke
- asparagus
- aubergine
- beetroot
- bok choi
- broccoli
- Brussels sprouts
- cabbage
- carrots
- cauliflower
- celeriac
- celery
- courgette
- cucumber
- endive
- fennel
- garlic
- kale
- leeks
- lettuce (any green leaf)
- mushroom
- okra
- olives
- onions
- parsnip
- peppers (all colours)
- pumpkin
- radish
- rocket
- spinach
- spring green
- spring onions
- squash
- swede
- sweet potato (no more than a fist-sized amount as part of your one-a-day carb portion)
- Swiss chard
- tomato
- turnips
- watercress

## Sea vegetables

Sea vegetables like samphire and seaweeds are extremely rich in minerals and a great way to boost your intake of good nutrients. You can cook samphire in boiling water for a few minutes and it goes really well with fish. With seaweed, don't go mad – just a sprinkle will do. It contains high levels of iodine, which can disrupt the function of the thyroid gland and in turn could have a detrimental effect on your weight-loss journey and general health.

## Nuts and seeds

Good as an occasional snack but not to eat in abundance if you want to lose weight. The rule of thumb is a small handful in food or as a snack once a day. Or use them as a garnish to scatter over your salads or other meals to add texture and crunch.

Types of nuts and seeds to include:

- almonds
- Brazil nuts
- chia seeds
- hazelnuts
- hemp seeds
- linseeds
- macadamias
- nut butters (except peanut)
- pecans
- pine nuts
- pistachios
- pumpkin seeds
- sesame seeds
- sunflower seeds
- walnuts

## Herbs and spices

Herbs and spices are very dense in nutrients. They support your immune system and give amazing flavours to your food. Use them in abundance when you're dieting as they can make seemingly bland food taste delicious with layers of flavour. You can eat chicken four days a week and it can taste totally different each time depending on the herbs and spices you add to it and how you cook it.

Types of herbs and spices to include: all kinds.

## Healthy fats and oils

Good oils and fats are essential for a healthy diet. They are also an excellent way to boost your omega-3 intake.

Types of oil to include:

- almond butter
- avocado oil
- coconut butter
- coconut oil (it's high in saturated fats, which you'll have heard are bad for you, but don't worry: the saturated fats contain MCT – medium chain triglycerides – are thought to actually give your metabolism a boost)
- lard (in moderation only as it's saturated, but that's great for cooking as saturated fats don't oxidize unhealthily when heated)
- macadamia oil
- olive oil
- unprocessed palm oil
- pumpkin seed butter
- rapeseed oil
- sesame oil
- tahini
- walnut oil
- any other naturally occurring oils from nuts and seeds

## Store cupboard and fridge basics

If you love milk in your tea, almond milk is a good substitute for dairy and agave and maple syrup are perfect healthy sweeteners instead of sugar. You'll find coconut yogurt is just as nice as cow's milk yogurt and the other ingredients will come in handy for making the puddings I'm going to show you in the next chapter.

- agave syrup or nectar (organic)
- ground almonds
- almond milk
- apple cider vinegar
- raw cacao powder
- chocolate nibs
- coconut flour
- coconut milk
- coconut yogurt
- coffee (beans)
- raw organic honey
- good grade maple syrup (organic)

- tamari
- tea (leaves)
- stevia (a natural, sugar-free sweetener)
- vanilla extract
- Xylitol (a natural, sugar-free sweetener)

### Grains

Not all grains are created equal. Make sure the grains you buy are as close to their natural state as possible and remember to cook and eat sparingly. I eat them as part of one meal every other day with a portion size equal to half a cup (64g) when uncooked. If you prefer not to measure, make sure it's no more than the size of your balled fist when cooked.

Types of grain to include:
- amaranth
- whole grain wheat and rye breads
- brown rice
- buckwheat
- millet
- oats and porridge
- wholewheat pasta
- quinoa
- spelt

## NO-GO FOODS

Below is a list of the foods you really should try and steer clear of, or cut back significantly.

*Any refined (white) or processed grain foods, particularly:*
- biscuits
- breakfast cereals with added sugar or not labelled as whole grain

- white bread and bagels
- cakes
- corn
- corn syrup
- crackers
- crumpets
- maize/corn flakes or savoury snacks
- muffins
- white pasta
- white rice
- wheat
- any flour, noodle or other food made out of any of these

### Legumes

Pulses get a thumbs up in official government healthy guidelines, and it's true that they are filling, high fibre and low fat, but to tell you the truth I'm not a big fan. Let me tell you why – I think that if you're already including healthy grains it's not wise to add extra carbohydrates, after all carbs are not are not a particular friend when you're trying to lose weight.

People with sensitive insides can also suffer significant gut issues with pulses (wind, diarrhoea and/or constipation, not to put too fine a point on it) as they're a high FODMAP food group (FODMAP stands for fermentable oligo-, di- and mono-saccharides and polyols and no, I'm not swearing). Research has found that in people who have irritable bowel syndrome (that's one in five of us at some time during our lives) turfing FODMAPs out of the diet can produce a significant reduction in symptoms.

Some researchers have also suggested that natural plant substances called lectins in pulses might not be very good if you're prone to autoimmune conditions like rheumatoid arthritis. The theory goes that if you've already been abusing your gut a bit with crap food (that was me by the way) these lectins can react with your intestines making them a bit 'leaky' and allowing allergens to pass through into your circulation which can result in a whole host of other problems. Fresh peas and green beans are included here as they are legumes but since they have lower levels of lectins and we don't usually eat them in large quantities some people think they are OK in moderation.

All this is a bit tentative and if you love your beans and pulses, never have any gut issues and find that they fill you up, go ahead. But my advice, while you're trying hard to whittle that waist and de-lard that derrière, is to include either a portion of whole grains or pulses, not both. A bit further down the road, when I'm sure my system has sorted itself completely and recovered from the rubbish I threw at it for years, I might stick a few beans on my whole grain toast, but until then I'm keeping them off the menu.

Types to avoid:

- adzuki beans
- broad beans
- butterbeans
- green beans
- horse beans
- kidney beans
- lima beans
- mung beans
- navy beans
- pinto beans
- red beans
- string beans
- white beans
- chickpeas
- lentils
- lupins
- mange tout (also called snowpea or sugar snap pea)
- mesquite
- miso
- peas
- peanuts (yes they are a legume not a nut!)
- soyabeans
- all soyabean products and derivatives
- tofu

### Refined sugar and sweeteners

- refined honey (OK in moderation)
- refined maple syrup
- brown sugar
- white sugar and all variants of processed sugars
- aspartame
- sucralose
- NutraSweet
- Splenda
- plus any other refined or man-made sweetener

### Drinks

Avoid all processed drinks, which means anything in a can or bottle that's not water. Full-fat or diet fizzy drinks or processed juice drinks are full of sugars and chemicals. Tea and coffee are OK.

### Oils and other store-cupboard ingredients

Try and avoid the following as far as possible:

- fruit juice – unless it comes straight from your juicer at home
- ketchup, chutneys and jams which contain sugar
- highly processed oils: any oil that is hydrogenated, partially hydrogenated, fractionated, refined or otherwise adulterated.
- most vegetable oils: any oil with a high omega-6 content that comes from a seed, grain or legume, such as corn, soyabeans, sunflower, safflower, cottonseed, grape seed, peanut and others. Rapeseed oil is okay as it's got some omega-3 to balance it. Omega-6 is a fatty acid and, while we do need some, the typical Western diet contains too much these days and it may increase your risk of heart disease.
- refined, iodized salt: use Himalayan sea salt or, better still, season with herbs, spices or pepper

Sticking to this list of foods works wonders for me. I have plenty of energy, am rarely hungry and don't have to sacrifice any flavours or foods I love. There's lots of research going on into the benefits of food, so let me tell you about a few superfoods, just to give you an idea of why this way of eating is so important – not only to lose weight, but also for our long-term health.

## THE SUPERFOODS

What makes a food a superfood? Well, we all know what makes a supermodel a supermodel, and it's the same for foods – they're the foods that deliver the most nutritious bang for their buck, the foods that literally have superpowers for health. They're dense in nutrition and carry amazing minerals and vitamins into your body, making you feel better by nourishing your body in ways that only Mother Nature can. Here are ten superfoods to include in your diet:

### 1. Spinach

Look no further than Popeye's big bulging muscles for a reason we should eat more of the green stuff. Spinach is a super green and it's bursting with vitamins A, C and K, plus magnesium and iron. Spinach contains a pile of antioxidants, which form part of the body's defence against the nasty cell changes that can lead to cancer. It has anti-inflammatory properties, great for when you're starting your workout programme. It's amazing for your vision, especially for age-related macular degeneration, and wonderful for your skin and bones (it's got more calcium than milk) and helps brain and liver function. Try eating raw or cooked spinach at least two or three times a week with meals.

## 2. Watercress

This is considered an anti-ageing food. Watercress is dense in vitamins A, B1, B2, B6, C, E and K among a whole load of others, which means this humble green supports a lot of your body's functions, as well as improving general health in structures like bones and teeth, your immune system, blood and memory. Eaten regularly, watercress contributes to good skin, hair and nails. Not keen on cabbage? Try watercress instead – it belongs to the same cruciferous family with anti-cancer benefits.

## 3. Blueberries

Blueberries are not only delicious, they also contain some lovely purple antioxidants called anthocyanins, which help keep skin and arteries firm and flexible, and blood pressure normal. As if that isn't enough, they also help your body battle against Alzheimer's and brain degeneration, as well as heart disease and various cancers.

## 4. Kale

Now, a lot of people haven't got to grips with kale yet, but let me tell you it is *packed* with good stuff. Rich in vitamins A, C, K, calcium, iron, folic acid and fibre, it's a great boost to your system, helping to lower blood pressure and reduce the risk of heart disease. It's also a strong antioxidant. No veg (apart from lovely spinach) comes close for its content of lutein, which helps protect the back of the eye from UV damage. Try a bag of kale drizzled with a teaspoon of olive oil and a couple of grinds of salt roasted in the oven for 15 minutes.

### 5. Chia seeds

These trendy little seeds are hot right now because they are an amazing combination, containing great omega-3s found in fish and nuts but also high in protein. Just one tablespoon provides around an eighth of the recommended daily allowance (RDA) of calcium and a sixth of the RDA of magnesium, so you couldn't get a better superfood for your bones. The seeds also aid weight-loss as they turn into a thick gel when mixed with water, making you feel fuller for longer. A study in the *Journal of Nutrition* found that a diet that included chia, soy and oats reduced glucose intolerance in susceptible patients, while another study in *Diabetes Care* found chia improved cardiovascular risk factors in type 2 diabetes. Try dipping a chicken breast in egg, rolling it in chia seeds and then frying it in some coconut oil until crispy on both sides.

### 6. Mackerel

This pretty little silvery fish is the top source of omega-3s and a good source of protein. It's packed with vitamins and minerals and will help protect your immune system. In addition to tasting great on the barbecue, it's packed with fatty acids that can help your body fight against various cancers too. And it's cheap as chips because it's so abundant.

### 7. Sweet potato

This great potato is not only delicious, it's also far more nutritious than normal potatoes and contains a good level of vitamins A, C and E, along with a host of others. Sweet potatoes release their energy more slowly than normal spuds, giving steadier blood-sugar levels. They're great to ward off illness, support your immune system and they're also packed with the anti-stress mineral magnesium, which helps heart health, muscle regeneration and the nervous function.

They're fab roasted, baked, grilled, poached, mashed, wedged and chipped. I eat up to a fist-sized portion at least three times a week.

## 8. Quinoa (pronounced 'keen-waa' )

This superfood has been popular for a few years now. Quinoa looks like a grain but is actually a seed rich in carbs and protein, whereas most grains are low in protein, so this is a great way to gain more nutrition from meals. High in magnesium, it will help reduce stress levels, plus it's also low in fat and offers a wide range of anti-inflammatory properties. Use this instead of couscous or rice – though once again you need to keep the portion small at 65g uncooked – or check out my porridge recipe on page 129 for a breakfast that will leave you feeling full until way after lunch.

## 9. Avocado

Whether it's in guacamole, as an alternative to butter, as a vegan or veggie protein source, grilled, mashed, stuffed, in salsa or made into chocolate mousse, avocado rocks. Avocadoes are one of a small number of crossover foods that can be used happily in both sweet and savoury dishes. This lovely little green pear is great for health; although it's high in fats, they're the good fats, and unlike most fruits and veg it also contains more than just a negligible bit of protein to add into the mix. They are rich in fibre, support your body's metabolism and condition the skin. Avocados are also one of the best sources of the antioxidant vitamin E. They promote heart and lung health and are packed with anti-inflammatory properties. They're also great at balancing out blood-sugar levels, and have anti-cancer properties to boot. Use them, but don't abuse them – twice a week in any of these forms is enough.

### 10. *Bananas*

Bananas are not hot food news right now but they should be, as they're an amazing food source and perfect for an energy boost. Containing vitamins B6 and C and high in magnesium, fibre and potassium, they offer protection against the risk of strokes and bone degeneration, they help your kidneys function well and are known to ease depression and stimulate serotonin to make you feel happier. Whether it's as a sugar substitute, mashed up hot or cold, a snack, a smoothie, frozen into a lolly, barbecued or dipped in dark chocolate, the humble banana is at home in almost every cooking environment you can think of. Bananas are high in natural sugars, so try to eat them early in the day and in moderation. These yellow lovelies are a perfect pre-workout snack because they're packed with energy. This delicious fruit is a great alternative if you're craving sugar.

## MULTITASKING INGREDIENTS

Superfoods are literally that: super. But there are other foods which I like to call multitaskers. These little blighters perform several functions at once, rather like most mums do. Here are my two favourites:

### *Coconut*

Coconut is the bomb. The main reason this tropical nut is the Swiss Army knife of ingredients is because there are massive health benefits to be gained from all its forms. The oil can sustain high temperatures without breaking down, so it's great for cooking, roasting and frying. The coconut itself is 90 per cent saturated fat, but it's a healthy kind and much less likely than the bad kind to be stored as fat in the body. The milk and cream is delicious in most foods and drinks, the coconut butter can be used instead of peanut butter, and all these forms deliver amazing benefits for your hair, skin and energy. Plus coconut is reckoned to be an appetite inhibitor, which means when you eat it you feel full for longer. It boosts brain function to boot. Use it sparingly, though: it won't help your waistline if you have too much.

## Almonds

A great low-fat nutty snack, but you can also try swapping peanut butter for organic almond butter – it has much less fat and far more benefits for the new you. Almond milk is also a winner: this tasty milk is delicious used to make porridge and a great alternative to dairy in a whole host of recipes. Try my almond blondies on page 176. Almonds also reduce cholesterol and your risk of heart and lung diseases and diabetes. A handful of almonds will also lower your risk of weight-gain, as they make you feel full very fast. As if that weren't enough, they also increase your energy levels.

# Weeks 1 and 2

Now you're ready to start, I'm going to share one of my top tips. First making sure the curtains are drawn or your nets are down – let's not put the neighbours off their grub – eat your next meal in front of the mirror in your undies or a bikini. I put a huge mirror in my dining room parallel with my dining table and ate at least one meal a day in a bikini for the first few weeks of my weight-loss journey. I was more than a bit chilly at times and I swear my Lukey thought I'd lost the plot. But I promise you, nothing will stop you overeating more than seeing your bare thighs, bum and belly while you chow down. Eating in the buff will sate even the hungriest of appetites in a heartbeat. I'm not encouraging anyone to go to extreme lengths, but eating in a bikini helped me become aware of just how much I was overeating at every meal when I didn't need to. Seeing the size of my waist and thighs while I was shoving dinner down my neck helped me realize that the volume of food I'd been used to eating had contributed to the size I hated. I learned to eat more slowly and stop the minute I was full because I was eating with my bits out.

Another tip is to make sure you never go hungry. Sometimes I'm not as organized as I'd like to be, but I try to make sure I always have something quick and simple in the fridge and freezer, even if it's just a marinade to chuck on a chicken breast before I roast it. And I always have good snacks on hand. I'm still tempted by that freshly baked bread smell in supermarkets, and there are days I'd love to smash my face into a croissant, but keeping quick tasty snacks like nuts or raw veggies around helps reduce the temptation.

If you're not constantly sated you're more likely to give in when a craving strikes. There are lots of tips on dealing with cravings in Chapter 9.

The recipes are in the next chapter and you can mix them up however you want. But if you don't fancy being creative after a workout session, I've done the hard work for you by setting out meal plans for the first two weeks. These meals mostly don't include extra carbs on the side. You can include one portion of whole grains or sweet potato a day and still lose weight but you will lose more if you cut them out completely. I haven't allowed for treat days on these meal plans but of course you can add one in.

## DAY 1

*breakfast*

- 1 slice of toasted rye bread, scrambled eggs and smoked salmon with watercress (eggs means 2 whole eggs; salmon 1 large slice)

*lunch*

- Chinese Chilli Pork Salad (pages 146–7)

*dinner*

- Breathe-Easy Thyme and Lemon BBQ Crust Chicken Cold Buster (page 153)

*dessert*

- Forever Young Vanilla Roasted Peaches (pages 179–80)

# DAY 2

*breakfast*

- The Grill Up: 1 rasher of bacon, 1 sausage, 1 tomato, 1 mushroom, 1 egg

*lunch*

- Hearty Happy Roasted Butternut Squash Soup (pages 138–9)

*dinner*

- Asian Bad Ass Sea Bass (pages 162–3)

# DAY 3

*breakfast*

- Homemade Nut Granola (pages 131–2)

*lunch*

- The Amazing Omelette (use 2 eggs) and green-leaf salad. Choose your omelette filling from: chicken and mushroom, bacon and tomatoes, salmon and asparagus, prawn and spring onion, mushroom and peppers, spinach and smoked salmon, ham and mushroom, prawn and red chilli, red onion and sweet potatoes, sliced steak and onion, turkey and cranberry, pork and apple, seafood and watercress. This meal is a great one to have a few times a week. It's easy, cheap and takes minutes to make. Find your favourite combo!

*dinner*

- Chinese Five Spiced Beef Energy Boost (pages 170–1)

*dessert*

- Choc 'o' Nuts Bar (pages 182–3)

## DAY 4

*breakfast*

- Poached eggs with spinach and mushrooms: poach 2 eggs and pan fry 4 sliced chestnut mushrooms and 2 handfuls spinach

*lunch*

- Crispy Salmon with Rocket Salad and Tamari Dressing (pages 134–5)

*dinner*

- I Heart Pork and Apricot Skewers (page 165)

## DAY 5

*breakfast*

- Fat Burning Banana and Bacon Pancakes (pages 130–1)

*lunch*

- Pork and Poached Egg Spinach and Squash Salad (pages 135–6)

*dinner*

- Lamb or Beef with Crunchy Coleslaw and Mustard Mayo (pages 154–5)

*dessert*

- Flourless Almond Butter Chocolate Chip Blondie (page 176)

## DAY 6

*breakfast*

- Omelette (use 2 eggs) with added cooked or smoked salmon pieces and some steamed asparagus spears cut into bite-sized pieces

*lunch*

- Face Lift Mango and Watercress Iron Power Salad (pages 147–8)

*dinner*

- Beefy Stuffed Peppers (pages 156–7)

## DAY 7

*breakfast*

- Skin Conditioning Coconut and Banana Cold Porridge (page 128)

*lunch*

- Super Smoking Mackerel Salad (pages 139–40)

*dinner*

- Moroccan Lemon Chicken Thighs (pages 157–8)

*dessert*

- Banana and Almond Lolly (page 175)

## DAY 8

*breakfast*

- Fresh berries and nuts, for example: 6 strawberries, small handful blueberries, 6 raspberries. 4 pecans, 4 macadamia nuts, 1 tablespoon pumpkin seeds, drizzle flax seed oil

*lunch*

- Maple Chicken Drummers (page 137)

*dinner*

- Energy and Iron Boosting Calf's Liver with Sweet Potato Mash (pages 160–1)

## DAY 9

*breakfast*

- Hot Mashed Banana and Pecans (page 127)

*lunch*

- Minute steak with mushrooms and beef tomato

*dinner*

- Lemon and Fennel Cod (pages 166–7)

*dessert*

- Choc 'O' Nut Bar (pages 182–3)

# DAY 10

*breakfast*

- Creamy Spicy Quinoa Porridge (page 129)

*lunch*

- Easy Chuck-In Chicken Stew (pages 143–4)

*dinner*

- Salmon with Avocado and Mango Salsa (page 159)

# DAY 11

*breakfast*

- Flash fry some steak (285g) with spinach and poached egg

*lunch*

- Face Lift and Body Repair Power Salad (page 133)

*dinner*

- Magic Trout Pout Protein Bake (pages 163–4)

*dessert*

- Avocado Chocolate Pudding (pages 177)

## DAY 12

*breakfast*

- Fresh fruit plate: a handful size each of banana, peach and melon with a handful of seeds (sunflower, sesame and pumpkin) and a dusting of cinnamon on top

*lunch*

- Prawn, Avocado and Bacon salad (page 149)

*dinner*

- Fillet Steak with Sweet Potato Wedges and Herby Sauce (pages 168–9)


## DAY 13

*breakfast*

- 2 rashers of bacon and a tomato

*lunch*

- Grilled Avocado and Peachy Salad (pages 145–6)

*dinner*

- Chocolate and Iron Up Beef Stew (pages 167–8)

*dessert*

- Mood-lifting BBQ Fruit Kebabs and Dipping Chocolate (pages 181–2)

# DAY 14

*breakfast*

- Fillet of smoked haddock, poached egg and spinach

*lunch*

- Asparagus with Poached Duck Egg and Fresh Dill Mayo (pages 142–3)

*dinner*

- Skinny Moussaka (pages 151–2)

# The Recipes

Over the next few pages I'm going to share some tried and tested recipes with you so you can get started today. Some of the ingredients may not be up your street, but don't let that put you off. It's all about substituting. Don't like prawns? Swap them for chicken breast. Don't fancy butternut squash? Switch it for sweet potato or pumpkin. Find your own rhythm and you're far more likely to stick to an eating plan.

The recipes are designed for the likes of me. When I first started out, I couldn't even boil an egg and thought poaching was when you trapped a wild animal. If you're like I used to be and the recipes on pages 127–83 seem a little daunting, start off with some of the 'Foods that Can Go Five Ways' on pages 185–9. These are tasty and easy meals with five different key ingredients that can be swapped in and out as you please – handy to keep in mind after a busy day or tiring weekend.

Just one thing to note: when the recipes call for salt and pepper, I would advise using sea salt, Celtic or Himalayan salt and freshly cracked black pepper for the best results. And for salad dressings, extra virgin olive oil has more flavour so I always use that.

# Beautiful Breakfasts

## HOT MASHED BANANA AND PECANS

*Serves 1*
*Prep 5 mins*
*Cook 5 mins*

1 tsp coconut butter
1 mashed banana
pinch cinnamon
pinch salt
25g pecans
25g blueberries

1. Warm the coconut butter gently in a pan and add the mashed banana.
2. Mix until heated through, add the cinnamon and salt and stir well.
3. Serve in a bowl sprinkled with the pecans and blueberries.

The Rules: You'll probably need a big banana for this, and don't let the mixture burn – just warm over a low heat.

The Goodness: Coconut oil in small amounts is great for your skin and hair. It also helps you shed excess fat as it contains good fats, which help you feel fuller for longer when eaten in moderation.

# SKIN CONDITIONING COCONUT AND BANANA COLD PORRIDGE

*Makes 4 servings*
*Prep 10 mins*

200g rolled oats
600ml coconut milk
2 tbsp agave syrup
2 bananas
sliced banana (to serve)
4 tbsp pecans, crushed

1. Place the oats and coconut milk in a bowl with the agave and mix, then cover and put in the fridge overnight.
2. Remove from fridge and blend in the bananas with a stick blender.
3. Serve nice and cold with an extra drizzle of agave and some sliced banana and crushed pecans.

The Rules: Make sure the mixture is covered when you chill it overnight, as otherwise the oats will absorb all the milk and then any other flavours you've got in the fridge. Garlic porridge? No thanks.

The Goodness: This is a brilliant breakfast and really delicious. Oats are a low glycaemic index food, which means they release energy slowly rather than all at once like a chocolate bar, so they keep you feeling fuller for longer. If you want to make this lower in fat content or find this mix too rich, replace half the coconut milk with water. Coconut milk is great for energy and for conditioning the skin, hair and nails.

# CREAMY SPICY QUINOA PORRIDGE

*Serves 2*
*Prep 10 mins*
*Cook 15 mins*

225g quinoa
120ml full-fat coconut milk
2 tbsp coconut sugar or agave (or plant-based sweetener of choice, such as honey or maple syrup)
pinch ground cardamom (optional)
pinch ground cinnamon (optional)
1 tbsp pecans or walnuts, crushed
¼ tbsp goji berries

1. Rinse the quinoa really well in a fine sieve.
2. Place the quinoa in a small pan with the coconut milk, 120ml water, coconut sugar or agave and spices (if you are using them), and bring to a simmer over high heat.
3. Reduce to a low heat and cover. Cook for 12–15 minutes.
4. Serve with the pecans or walnuts and goji berries on top, or your preferred blend of nuts and dried fruit.

The Rules: If you're looking for an alternative to oats, this is perfect. Mix it up a bit by trying different combinations of toppings, like almond and banana, apricot and pumpkin seeds, or hazelnuts and dried cherries. Use fresh or dried fruit (but go lightly on the dried fruit – it's high in sugars).

The Goodness: Quinoa is a great alternative to oats and couscous. It's a seed and therefore naturally higher in protein and kinder to the digestive system.

# FAT BURNING BANANA AND BACON PANCAKES

*Serves 2*
*Prep 5 mins*
*Cook 10 mins*

1 banana
1 egg
8g (1 tbsp) ground almonds
8g (1 tbsp) coconut flour
pinch salt
pinch cinnamon
1 rasher lean bacon
sliced banana (to serve)
1 red chilli, finely chopped
honey or good grade maple syrup

1. Mash up, mix or (even better) put in a blender the banana, egg, ground almonds, coconut flour, salt and cinnamon, and whizz until it's smoothie consistency. Add a splash of water if the mixture is too thick.
2. Grill lean bacon until crispy – about 4 minutes.
3. Heat a non-stick pan. Pour three small amounts of pancake mix (each about the size of a biscuit) into the pan. Cook until the underside gets golden brown, then flip the pancakes and cook the other side until golden.
4. Stack the pancakes on a plate and serve with crispy bacon and sliced banana on the side. Scatter the red chilli over the plate, then add a small drizzle of honey or maple syrup.

The Rules: Go easy on the honey or maple syrup – literally just a small drizzle is enough.

The Goodness: Bananas are a great source of potassium, which supports your heart, and vitamin B6, which is great for your blood. Chilli speeds the metabolism.

---

## HOMEMADE NUT GRANOLA

*Makes 10 servings*
*Prep 10 mins*
*Cook 20 mins*

100g almonds, hazelnuts, macadamia and Brazil nuts
100g dried plums, cherries, cranberries or apricots
50g pumpkin seeds
50g ground almonds
50g desiccated coconut, unsweetened
50g coconut flakes (optional)
25g chia seeds
75g coconut oil, melted
1 tbsp good-quality manuka honey
splash vanilla extract
zest of 1 orange

1. Preheat oven to 165°C/gas 3.
2. Place the whole nuts and dried fruit in a food processor. Grind the mixture into medium-sized crumbs: some of it will turn into a finer flour-like consistency and some of it will stay chunky – a mix of the two is perfect. You can break up the nuts and fruit in a pestle and mortar if you don't have a food processor.
3. Pour the mixture into a large mixing bowl and add all the other

ingredients. Get your hands in to mix together all the dry and wet ingredients – it'll look a right mess, but don't worry.

4. Line a roasting tray with baking paper, making sure the sides are covered, otherwise it'll stick. Spoon the mixture into a tray and spread it out.

5. Bake for 10 minutes in the oven, then take out and carefully mix it up a bit so all the granola gets golden and crunchy. Spread it out again and bake for another 10 minutes, then take out to cool for 30 minutes. Put it in the fridge for an hour so the coconut oil fully sets.

6. Crumble it up and store in an airtight container. It should keep well for about 10 days.

The Rules: If you're a granola fan, aim to eat this two or three times a week only, as it's a lot of nuts to eat every day.

The Goodness: This is rich in omega-3 fatty acids, great for heart health, boosting your immune system and reducing inflammation.

# Lush Lunches

## FACE LIFT AND BODY REPAIR POWER SALAD

*Serves 1*
*Prep 10 mins*
*Cook 20 mins*

1 egg
100g watercress
20g red onion, finely sliced
1 avocado, sliced
extra virgin olive oil
pinch chilli flakes

1. Heat a pan of water to boiling and cook your egg for 3–4 minutes (4 if you want it hard boiled). Leave to cool and then peel and slice.
2. Mix the watercress with the red onion and pile on a plate. Add the sliced avocado and egg, then drizzle with a little olive oil and dust with the chilli flakes. Season with salt and pepper.

The Rules: Go easy on the oil and salt and pepper – they are there to add delicate flavour, not for whacking on.

The Goodness: Watercress contains massive amounts of vitamin C and is great for energy levels; eat it every day if possible. Eggs and avocado do wonders to help balance your energy and mood levels. They're packed with protein to keep you going and help your body rebuild itself after injury or exertion.

# CRISPY SALMON WITH ROCKET SALAD AND TAMARI DRESSING

*Serves 1*
*Prep 10 mins*
*Cook 20 mins*

coconut oil
130g salmon fillet
1 tsp coconut flour
50g rocket
¼ red onion, finely sliced
half a tomato
small handful cashew nuts
¼ avocado, sliced
1 lemon

*Dressing*
1 tbsp tamari (wheat-free soy sauce)
1 tbsp olive oil
1 tsp Dijon mustard
1 clove garlic, crushed
1 tsp chopped ginger

1. Preheat oven to 160°C/gas 3.
2. To make the dressing, mix together the tamari, olive oil, mustard, garlic and ginger in a small bowl and leave to stand.
3. Heat a non-stick pan over a high heat and add a tiny amount of coconut oil. Place the salmon skin side down into a saucer of coconut flour, dust off excess and fry for 2 minutes or until golden and remove from pan.
4. Place the salmon skin side up on a baking tray lined with baking

parchment and cook in the oven for a further 10 minutes or until firm to touch. Remove from oven and allow to rest for a few minutes.

5. Mix together the rocket, onion, tomato, cashews and avocado in a bowl and drizzle with half the dressing, then pile in the middle of a plate. Place the salmon on top and drizzle again with the rest of the dressing and add a squeeze of lemon juice. Lush!

The Rules: Tamari is wheat and gluten free; but it still has a high salt content, so use sparingly.

The Goodness: Salmon is an excellent source of protein and fat, rich in omega-3 and vitamin D.

----

## PORK AND POACHED EGG SPINACH AND SQUASH SALAD

*Serves 1*
*Prep 15 mins*
*Cook 30 mins*

150g good-quality pork sausage meat
¼ butternut squash, peeled
apple cider vinegar
pinch salt
1 egg
2 handfuls spinach

1. Roll 4 small balls of sausage meat and place under a hot grill for 20 minutes, turning occasionally.

2. Chop the squash into small pieces and add under the grill next to the pork to cook at the same time.
3. Heat a pan of water until boiling and add a splash of vinegar and a pinch of salt. Stir water into a whirlpool and crack the egg into the water. Poach for 2–3 minutes maximum, until the white is set.
4. When the pork and squash are cooked, remove from the grill. If they're cooked you will be able to slide a butter knife into the squash chunks and the pork will be firm to the touch. Put the squash and sausages in a bowl with the spinach and mix it all together with your hands so that the flavours start to fuse. Then add the poached egg on top, cut in half so that the yolk drips onto the other ingredients, and season with salt and pepper.

The Rules: Make sure your pork and eggs are good quality – go organic if you can.

The Goodness: Spinach is amazing for your eyesight and jam-packed with vitamin B9 and folic acid, which are great for healthy blood cells, as well as magnesium, calcium and iron. Spinach is a nutrient-dense superfood and should be eaten as often as possible.

# MAPLE CHICKEN DRUMMERS

*Serves 4*
*Prep 10 mins*
*Cook 40 mins*

Sesame oil
8 good-quality chicken drumsticks
maple syrup
300g bacon lardons or chopped smoked bacon
80g pecan nuts, crushed
1 lemon
100g watercress

1. Preheat oven to 200°C/gas 6. Add a drizzle of sesame oil to a baking tray and add the drumsticks. Cover the drumsticks with a good drizzle of maple syrup. Cook for 10 minutes, turning halfway.
2. Remove the drumsticks from the tray and add the bacon and pecans, then sprinkle the zest and juice of the lemon all over the top. Carefully mix everything together, put the chicken back on top and return to the oven for 20–30 minutes until the chicken is golden, sticky and cooked through.
3. Serve on a large dish with a watercress salad and season to taste.

The Rules: The drummers also keep well in the fridge for snacking on.

The Goodness: Chicken is a great source of lean protein, while watercress is a great source of iron, vitamin A and vitamin C.

# HEARTY HAPPY ROASTED BUTTERNUT SQUASH SOUP

*Serves 4*
*Prep 15 mins*
*Cook 90 mins*

1 large butternut squash
olive oil
1 sprig thyme
pinch chilli flakes
1 tsp turmeric
1 tsp cumin seeds
3 cloves garlic
1 white onion
850ml vegetable broth or chicken stock
120g cashew nuts

1. Preheat the oven to a medium-high temperature: about 175°C–180°C/gas 4.
2. Slice the squash (with skin still on) in half and remove the seeded area, cut into rough chunks and place in a baking tray. Drizzle with olive oil and sprinkle over the thyme, chilli flakes, turmeric and cumin seeds, then season with salt and pepper and roast in the oven for around 30–45 minutes until the squash is golden and roasted. Leave to one side to cool before peeling.
3. Heat a splash of olive oil over a medium heat and sweat the garlic and onions until soft.
4. Add the peeled squash and cook for another 5 minutes.
5. Pour over the stock and simmer gently for 10 minutes.

6. Remove from heat and with a stick blender whizz together until it's a lovely thick consistency and all the chunks have been blended.
7. Toast the cashews in a hot dry pan and then crush them up.
8. Serve in a bowl with cashews sprinkled over the top, along with some fresh thyme and a drizzle of olive oil.

The Rules: Make this easy by roasting the squash with skin on and whacking everything in the oven.

The Goodness: Butternut squash is rich in dietary fibre and carotenoid antioxidants, which support your immune system.

---

## SUPER SMOKING MACKEREL SALAD

*Serves 4*
*Prep 10 mins*
*Cook 15 mins*

100g quinoa
1 tub goats yogurt or Greek yogurt
½ bunch mint, finely chopped
1 bunch asparagus (10–15 spears)
100g lamb's lettuce
100g red chard, chopped
4 fillets smoked mackerel
50g alfalfa
200g beetroot (cooked but not pickled), quartered
1 pomegranate, seeded

1. Rinse the quinoa well until the water runs clear and then put in a pan with 1 part quinoa to 2 parts water and bring to the boil. Cook for 10 minutes, then drain away any excess liquid and leave to the side covered with a lid. The grains should steam into a light fluffy mix.
2. Mix together the pot of yogurt with half of the mint.
3. Break the woody ends off the asparagus and lightly grill for 3–6 minutes, turning halfway, then leave to cool.
4. Mix the lamb's lettuce, chopped chard, quinoa and the rest of the mint together in a bowl and add a large handful to each plate.
5. Break each mackerel fillet down into chunks and scatter it evenly over each plate of salad. Add two or three asparagus spears, some beetroot and a handful of the pomegranate seeds. Top each with a handful of alfalfa sprouts, then drizzle over the mint and yogurt dressing and serve.

The Rules: Make sure the quinoa is cooked well and fluffy in texture – this won't happen if you forget to rinse it well at the start.

The Goodness: Mackerel is a superfood fish. It's packed with omega-3s and a marvellous boost for your skin and bones.

# ENERGY BOOSTER POWER SALAD

*Serves 1*
*Prep 10 mins*
*Cook 20 mins*

40g watercress
1 small beetroot, quartered
2 spring onions, finely sliced
½ cucumber, finely sliced
1 salmon fillet, approx. 100g, pre-cooked (or roast or grill a fresh
    fillet for 15–20 minutes)

*Dressing*
2 tsp Dijon mustard
1 orange
2 tbsp apple cider vinegar

1.  Mix together the watercress, beetroot, spring onion and cucumber in a bowl.
2.  For the dressing, mix the mustard, the juice of the orange and vinegar in a small bowl and season with salt and pepper. Make sure you mix well so the flavours can merge.
3.  Place the salad on a dish and drizzle with the dressing, then add the cooked salmon. Serve with a little orange zest on top.

The Rules: Balance out the dressing to your liking: taste it and adjust to make it sweeter or sharper to suit your palate.

The Goodness: Beetroot is bursting with liver-detoxifying properties, while salmon is a powerhouse of good fats, great protein and essential oils, amazing for supporting skin, eyes, hair and nails.

# ASPARAGUS WITH POACHED DUCK EGG AND FRESH DILL MAYO

*Serves 2*
*Prep 10 mins*
*Cook 10 mins*

2 egg yolks
apple cider vinegar
juice of ½ lemon
½ bunch fresh dill
extra virgin olive oil
1 bunch of asparagus (10–15 spears)
4 duck eggs

1.  To make the mayonnaise, whizz together 2 egg yolks, a splash of vinegar, the lemon juice and some chopped dill (about a handful) with a stick blender or in a food processor for 1 minute. Slowly add a running trickle of olive oil to the mix and keep blending until the mixture starts to change in consistency and get thick and paler yellow in colour. This usually takes 2–3 minutes. You can use a balloon whisk instead of a blender; it takes around 8 minutes whisking by hand.
2.  Half fill a pan with water, bring to the boil and place steaming pan on top.
3.  Break the woody ends off the asparagus and place in steaming pan for 3–5 minutes or until al dente (still a bit of crunch). Leave the pan simmering for you to poach the eggs.
4.  Now poach your eggs – duck eggs are slightly larger than chicken eggs, so they might take a while longer. Add a splash of vinegar to the pan of simmering water and stir around vigorously to

create a whirlpool. Crack eggs into pan and carefully stir around until the eggs are cooked – usually this will take 6–8 minutes depending on the size of the eggs.

5. Place about 6 spears of asparagus on each plate, add a big dollop of delicious mayonnaise, place the eggs on top and season with salt and pepper.

The Rules: This little veggie number tastes amazing. Make sure nothing gets overcooked. You can use chicken eggs too, of course, but duck eggs have a very distinct, delicious flavour and are lighter in consistency.

The Goodness: Duck eggs are packed with protein. They're higher in wonder vitamin D than chicken eggs and are a great source of B12. Asparagus is known for its very high levels of folic acid and it's packed with prebiotics, which boost the good bugs in your gut and your immune system too. It's a natural diuretic, meaning it helps take excess water and salts out of the body. It also tastes delicious and is dead easy to prepare.

---

## EASY CHUCK-IN CHICKEN STEW

*Serves 2*
*Prep 10 mins*
*Cook 30 mins*

1 carrot
2 sticks celery
½ white onion
¼ butternut squash
1 clove garlic

½ head of green cabbage or spring greens
1 chicken stock cube
4 chicken thighs, skinned
olive oil
1 tsp fresh thyme
pinch mixed herbs

1. Chop up all the vegetables into small chunks of about the same size, crush the garlic and finely shred the cabbage or greens.
2. Place pan on a medium heat and add a splash of olive oil, cook the garlic and onion for 30 seconds, then add the chicken thighs and fry off for 3–5 minutes until golden. Remove the meat from the pan and put to one side.
3. In the same pan, mix the stock cube with 1 pint of boiling water, then add all the rest of the chopped veg and herbs. Season with salt and pepper, put a lid on the pan and simmer for 15 minutes. When it's all cooked down, you may want to add another quarter-pint of water, depending on the consistency of the veg and how much liquid has evaporated. At this point, strip the chicken meat from the bones and add the meat to the pan.
4. Cook together for a further 10 minutes, then take the lid off and allow to cool for 10 minutes before serving in a deep soup bowl.

The Rules: Don't be tempted to find a big chunky piece of bread to dip in – this contains all you need to fill you up. You can also use turkey if you like.

The Goodness: A great little cheap pot of lean chicken protein and veggies packed with goodness, this meal will keep you full for a long time. It's low-fat comfort food that can be cooked in large batches in advance and frozen to save you time.

# GRILLED AVOCADO AND PEACHY SALAD

*Serves 4*
*Prep 10 mins*
*Cook 10 mins*

500g cherry tomatoes
1 bunch fresh basil, roughly torn
100g pea shoots
1 handful walnuts
balsamic vinegar
4 peaches
2 avocados
1 bag mixed leaves
extra virgin olive oil

1. Halve the tomatoes and place in bowl, then add the basil, pea shoots, walnuts and a splash of balsamic vinegar. Season with salt and pepper and mix together.
2. Heat a griddle pan to a high heat. Meanwhile cut the peaches and avocados into quarters and remove the stones and avocado peel.
3. Place the peach and avocado quarters on the griddle pan. To get those attractive chargrilled lines, leave each piece in the same place without moving for at least 2 minutes. Remove from the pan and leave to cool.
4. Put the leaves in a bowl, add the tomato mix and toss together. Place the peaches and avocado on top with another small drizzle of balsamic and extra virgin olive oil. Serve immediately.

The Rules: Be aware of the heat of the griddle: if it's not hot enough, food will stick and it's a nightmare to get off. The hotter the better, as you need to make sure you sear rather than fry food.

The Goodness: Avocado and peaches are great for the skin and packed with healthy fats.

---

## CHINESE CHILLI PORK SALAD

*Serves 4*
*Prep 20 mins*
*Cook 15 mins*

3 carrots
2 cucumbers
1 tbsp apple cider vinegar
2 tbsp agave syrup
3 limes
pinch salt
800g pork fillet
1 tbsp chilli sauce
1 bunch coriander, chopped
4 Chinese cabbage leaves
olive oil
4 skewers

1. Slice up the carrot and cucumber with a julienne shredder (like a potato peeler with rivets in to make spaghetti-like strands). If you don't have a shredder, just use a grater.
2. Mix together the vinegar, agave, the zest and juice of 1 lime,

and salt in a bowl, then add the carrot and cucumber strips and leave to marinate for 15 minutes.

3. Heat a griddle pan to a high heat and add a drizzle of olive oil. Meanwhile dice the pork fillet, put the cubes on skewers and drizzle over the chilli sauce.

4. Cook the pork for 3–5 minutes on each side. You want to keep the meat tender, so don't overcook it.

5. Place a Chinese cabbage leaf on each plate, cover with a handful of the cucumber and carrot mixture on top, then add the skewer on top. Garnish with coriander and 2 lime wedges.

The Rules: Don't overcook this lovely cut of pork – it's easy for the meat to become chewy and ruin the effect. Use a griddle pan or barbecue at a hot heat so the meat doesn't stick.

The Goodness: Raw veggies are an excellent source of nutrients (cooking can remove vitamin C in particular). Pork is a great source of protein and vitamin B1, which is needed for your cells to release energy.

---

# FACE LIFT MANGO AND WATERCRESS IRON POWER SALAD

*Serves 4*
*Prep 10 mins*

2 mangos
100g red cabbage
100g watercress
100g bean sprouts

½ bunch mint
1 red chilli, finely chopped
100g halved almonds, roughly chopped

*Dressing*
1 tbsp fish sauce
juice of 1 lime
1 tbsp tamari
olive oil

1. Chop the mango into 1cm chunks. Shred the red cabbage and soak in water for 1 hour.
2. Gently mix all the salad ingredients together in a bowl.
3. For the dressing, mix together the fish sauce, lime juice and tamari with a splash of olive oil. Lightly sprinkle over salad and serve.

The Rules: This is great eaten alone or as a side dish with white fish or meat; it suits everything from chicken to steak.

The Goodness: Watercress is a wonder. This amazing wrinkle-buster contains more vitamin C than oranges and more beta-carotene and vitamin A than apples, tomatoes and broccoli. It's absolutely packed with iron and has a delicious peppery taste. I eat it most days.

# PRAWN, AVOCADO AND BACON SALAD

*Serves 1*
*Prep 10 mins*
*Cook 5 mins*

1 rasher lean bacon
1 small cos lettuce
½ avocado
1 small tin sweetcorn
8 king prawns, precooked

*Dressing*
½ lemon
1 tbsp extra virgin olive oil
apple cider vinegar

1. Grill the bacon for 5 minutes and chop into small pieces.
2. Chop lettuce and avocado and place in a bowl, mix in the sweetcorn and bacon pieces, then lightly drizzle with extra virgin olive oil.
3. For the dressing, put the lemon juice, oil and a splash of vinegar in small bowl, season with salt and pepper and mix well.
4. Place the salad mix on a plate or in a bowl, lay the prawns on top and drizzle with dressing.

The Rules: Use good-quality prawns and buy precooked for ease and speed.

The Goodness: Prawns are a good source of protein, zinc and omega-3s.

# Delicious Dinners

## SKINNY MOUSSAKA

*Serves 4*
*Prep 10 mins*
*Cook 90 mins*

2 aubergines
olive oil
1 white onion, chopped
2 cloves garlic, crushed
500g lamb mince
2 plum tomatoes, chopped
1 tbsp tomato puree
1 tsp cinnamon
1 tsp finely grated nutmeg
1 bunch fresh parsley, chopped
400g baby spinach

1. Preheat the oven to 160°C/gas 3.
2. Slice the aubergines in half lengthways and place in a baking tray with an inch of water in the bottom, sprinkle over a little salt and cook in the oven for 20–30 minutes, turning them over halfway. Allow to cool but leave the oven on.
3. Heat a splash of olive oil in a deep pan and cook the onion and garlic for 1 minute. Add the lamb mince and sauté for another 5 minutes, then add the chopped tomatoes, tomato puree and the spices.

4. Meanwhile scoop out the cooled aubergine flesh, setting aside the skins, and add this to the lamb mix. Add half the parsley and simmer for 5 minutes.
5. Place the aubergine skins in a deep dish and spoon in the lamb mix, folding the aubergine skin over to create little parcels, and bake in the oven for an hour.
6. Allow to cool for 10 minutes and then serve on a bed of baby spinach.

The Rules: This is definitely a dish to make more of and freeze up. Only use good-quality lamb mince.

The Goodness: Cinnamon is known to help lower blood-sugar levels for diabetes sufferers. It's used a lot in Greek cooking and is one of my top 'super spices', along with turmeric.

Aubergines are one of my favourite vegetables, but they can be tricky to cook as they are very spongy and absorb oil and water very easily. Part of the nightshade family that also includes tomatoes, pepper and potatoes, they are high in fibre and magnesium, which massively supports the muscle and nervous system, helping to build strong bones. They're also packed with vitamin K, which helps protect against cancer and heart disease.

# BREATHE-EASY THYME AND LEMON BBQ CRUST CHICKEN COLD BUSTER

*Serves 2*
*Prep 10 mins*
*Cook 30 mins*

1 whole chicken (organic, or the best quality you can buy)
1 bunch fresh thyme leaves
4 lemons
4 cloves garlic, crushed

1. Ask your butcher to strip out and bone the chicken.
2. Mix together the thyme with the zest from all four lemons and the juice of two, plus the garlic and a little salt and pepper. Rub this mixture all over the chicken and leave in the fridge for 30 minutes – longer if possible.
3. Barbecue or grill the chicken whole for 20–30 minutes until crispy and golden on all sides, turning every 5 or 10 minutes. Let it rest for 10 minutes.
4. Chop into chunks that can be eaten by hand and serve with lemon wedges and sprigs of fresh thyme.

The Rules: This dish is a great for barbecue parties: it's easy to prepare and you can make up two chickens and cook then refrigerate – it's delicious served cold with a green salad.

The Goodness: This lovely dish is not only packed with lean protein, but the thyme also has healing properties and has been traditionally used to ease chest congestion and breathing problems.

# LAMB OR BEEF STEAK WITH CRUNCHY COLESLAW AND MUSTARD MAYO

*Serves 2*
*Prep 10 mins*
*Cook 20 mins*

450g good-quality lamb or beef steak
agave syrup
pinch cumin
pinch dill
pinch caraway seeds
apple cider vinegar
¼ small red cabbage
¼ small white cabbage
1 carrot
¼ onion

*Mayonnaise*
2 egg yolks
8–10 tbsp extra virgin olive oil
1 tsp Dijon mustard

1. Lightly grill the steak for 5–10 mins on either side, depending how you like it cooked, and leave it to rest before slicing thinly.
2. Mix a splash of agave with the cumin, dill and caraway seeds in a bowl and add a splash of the apple cider vinegar. Set aside so the flavours can infuse.
3. Using the grater or fine shredder setting on your food processor, whizz up the cabbage, carrot and onion. Alternatively finely slice the cabbage and onion and grate the carrot.
4. To make the mayo, whizz together the egg yolks with a stick

blender or a food processor. Slowly add a running trickle of olive oil to the mix and keep blending until the mixture starts to change in consistency and get thick, and a paler yellow in colour. This usually takes 2–3 minutes. You can use a balloon whisk in-stead of a blender; it takes around 8 minutes whisking by hand. Add the mustard and blend again for 15 seconds.

5. Place all the shredded veg into a bowl and mix together. Add the mayo and mix again, making sure it coats all the vegetables.

6. Place a good handful of the slaw on each plate and add half the steak. Add the mayo in a small dipping dish on the side before serving.

The Rules: Cook the steak to your preferred taste: if you like it cooked medium, it should be firm to the touch when it comes off the grill. Go lightly on the mayo – it's delicious but high in fats, so this is a treat!

The Goodness: Eating raw veggies gives you the full nutritional benefit of all the vitamin C in them, rather than killing it off by cooking.

# BEEFY STUFFED PEPPERS

*Serves 2*
*Prep 15 mins*
*Cook 30 mins*

olive oil
½ white onion, chopped
1 large clove garlic, crushed
1 tomato, chopped
1 400g tin chopped tomatoes
½ bunch fresh parsley, chopped
60g chopped walnuts
100g spinach, chopped
1 tsp smoked paprika
200g good-quality lean beef mince
1 red pepper

1. Preheat oven to 200°C/gas 6.
2. Heat a splash of olive oil in a pan and cook the onion and garlic for 5 minutes. When they start to soften and go see-through, add the fresh tomato, tinned tomatoes, parsley, walnuts, half the spinach and the paprika. Season with salt and pepper and sweat it down all together for about 5–10 minutes until reduced in volume.
3. Heat a separate pan and fry the beef mince in a tiny bit of oil for 5–8 minutes until it is half cooked and some of the meat fat has been brought out. Drain the fat off and add the meat to the tomato mixture, mix well and cook for a further 15 minutes. Leave to cool for 10 minutes.
4. Cut the pepper in half lengthways and lay the halves on a baking

tray. Spoon the mince mix inside each half, patting down as you go until they're totally full, then place in the oven for 15 minutes until the pepper is cooked.

5. Remove and allow to stand for 5 minutes. Serve on a bed of the rest of the spinach leaves.

The Rules: If you like this dish, you can double or even triple the quantities of the mince mix and freeze it down for the future – all you need to do is defrost it, add it to the peppers and cook. Double the amounts of the ingredients for four servings, triple for six servings, and so on. This dish is also delicious served cold.

The Goodness: Red peppers are packed with vitamin C and beta-carotene, which can be used by the body as an antioxidant or turned into vitamin A.

------

## MOROCCAN LEMON CHICKEN THIGHS

*Serves 2*
*Prep 10 minutes*
*Cook 20 mins*

¼ tsp turmeric
¼ tsp ginger
¼ tsp cumin
¼ tsp cinnamon
3 lemons
olive oil
4 chicken thighs (best quality you can afford)
570ml good-quality chicken stock

1 jar mixed pitted olives
1 bunch fresh thyme
200g mixed green leaves

1. Mix all the spices together with the juice of a lemon and rub this paste all over the chicken thighs. Leave to marinate for at least 30 minutes – preferably a few hours or overnight in the fridge.
2. Heat a splash of olive oil in a frying pan to a high heat, place chicken thighs in pan and sear until the skin or flesh is golden (about 1–3 minutes), then turn down heat.
3. Mix together the juice of another lemon, the chicken stock and 4 cups of water and add to the pan. Slice the remaining lemon and place on top of the chicken.
4. Add the olives and bunch of thyme, cover with a lid and cook for 10 minutes, then simmer gently with the lid off for 30 minutes.
5. Serve with the cooking juices drizzled over the top for a dressing and a small green salad.

The Rules: If losing weight is your top priority, it's better to skin the thighs before cooking. The skin should peel off easily if you pull it sharply away from the flesh; if in doubt, ask your butcher or meat counter to do it for you.

The Goodness: Turmeric has great anti-inflammation qualities and has been used for hundreds of years in Chinese and Indian medicine. Don't be shy about using this spice: it's got a fairly delicate flavour but is a truly an awesome ingredient.

# SALMON WITH AVOCADO AND MANGO SALSA

*Serves 4*
*Prep 5 mins*
*Cook 10 mins*

1 avocado, chopped
1 mango, chopped
½ red onion, chopped
½ red pepper, chopped
1 tbsp jalapeño peppers, chopped
½ bunch coriander
2 tbsp fresh lime juice
olive oil
4 salmon fillets

1.  Mix together the avocado, mango, red onion, red pepper, jalapeño peppers and lime juice. Add the chopped coriander, season with salt and pepper and lightly crush with a fork to release the juices of all the ingredients. Set aside in the fridge so the flavours fuse.
2.  Heat a splash of olive oil in a large pan over a medium-high heat. Season the salmon with salt and pepper and sear for 3 to 5 minutes on each side – start with the skin side down, cook until that's golden and then turn.
3.  Serve on a plate topped with a heaped spoon of delicious salsa.

The Rules: You can add more chilli and also some garlic to the salsa if you like for an extra kick!

The Goodness: This is an excellent dish for your skin: salmon is packed with amazing omega-3s and vitamins B and D. Avocado is rich in fibre and packed with vitamin E. These two ingredients are a great combo, helping you feel fuller for longer.

# ENERGY AND IRON BOOSTING CALF'S LIVER WITH SWEET POTATO MASH

*Serves 4*
*Prep 10 mins*
*Cook 30 mins*

4 sweet potatoes, peeled and cut into chunks
1 tbsp manuka honey
1 red chilli, chopped
½ bunch coriander
2 cloves garlic
olive oil
6 shallots
300ml beef stock
2 tbsp apple cider vinegar
1 tsp Dijon mustard
1 tsp arrowroot, dissolved in 1 tbsp water
1 tbsp ground almond flour or coconut flour
4 slices calf's liver, about 125g each
200g bag of spinach

1. Boil the sweet potatoes in a pan of lightly salted water for 15 minutes. Drain and mash well, then add the honey, chilli, half the coriander, 1 finely chopped garlic clove and a splash of olive oil and mix together. Cover with a lid to keep in the heat and put to one side.
2. Finely slice the shallots and the other garlic clove and fry in a splash of olive oil until golden and caramelized.
3. Add half of the beef stock, stir well and reduce the heat to a simmer, then add the vinegar, mustard and arrowroot to thicken.

Season with salt and pepper and continue to stir, adding the rest of the stock to make a nice thick gravy. Leave to one side.

4. Mix the almond or coconut flour with a little salt and pepper in a bowl and then coat the calf's liver in flour mix.

5. Heat a drizzle of olive oil in a pan to a high heat. Dust the excess flour from the liver and cook for about 1–3 minutes on each side (depending on thickness) until the meat is cooked through and golden brown on the outside but still pink inside.

6. In another pan, heat a couple of tablespoons of water to simmer then add the spinach and wilt quickly. It should take no longer than a minute or two – you still want it to be a vibrant green.

7. Serve a good spoon of the mash with a slice of calf's liver on top and some spinach to the side. Drizzle the gravy over the top and add some cracked black pepper.

The Rules: This has a few things going on for you to balance. Focus on the sauce: it will get thicker as it cools, so concentrate on getting this right. Also you want the liver to be tender – try not to overcook it or the meat will become tough. If you're not sure, cut a small piece off and fry it separately as a test, so that you can adjust cooking times accordingly.

The Goodness: This dish delivers a big punch of energy and iron. If I'm feeling exhausted, this is what I crave and it always sorts me out. The high content of iron from the liver and the spinach makes it a truly fantastic energy-boosting dish.

# ASIAN BAD ASS SEA BASS

*Serves 4*
*Prep 5 mins*
*Cook 10–20 mins*

4 sea bass fillets, around 125g each
2 shallots
2.5cm piece ginger
4 cloves garlic
2 red chillies
1 stick lemongrass
2 lemons
30ml tamari
sesame oil
apple cider vinegar
olive oil
1 bunch coriander
2 spring onions
4 radishes

1. Get your fishmonger to prepare the fish: ask him to remove the gut, head, fins, scales and tail. Chop each fish into 4 large chunks.
2. To make the Asian paste, whizz together in a blender the shallots, ginger, garlic, 1 chilli, lemongrass, juice of both lemons, tamari, a splash each of sesame oil, vinegar and olive oil, plus half the coriander until finely blended.
3. Finely slice the spring onion, radishes, the remaining chilli and rest of the coriander for the garnish.
4. Place the fish pieces in a large baking tray, pour over the Asian paste and mix carefully, making sure all the fish is coated,

then cover and place in the fridge for minimum of an hour to marinate – the longer the better.

5. Cook the fish pieces on a barbecue, or under a hot grill for 5–10 minutes, turning when the skin is golden and crispy.

6. Serve scattered with the spring onion, radish, chilli and coriander mix.

The Rules: Barbecuing will give this dish a lovely smoky flavour, but the fish will cook a lot faster on a barbecue, so be aware that it will only need a couple of minutes on each side.

The Goodness: Sea bass is a brilliant source of protein and contains good omega-3 fats. The ginger and garlic and all the typical Asian fresh ingredients offer numerous benefits for respiratory and skin health.

---

## MAGIC TROUT POUT PROTEIN BAKE

*Serves 4*
*Prep 10 mins*
*Cook 30 mins*

4 trout fillets, about 180g each
4 tbsp olive oil
200g cherry tomatoes (preferably on the vine)
1 tbsp capers
1 bunch parsley
1 clove garlic
200g mixed chargrilled vegetables (cook your own, or buy from the deli counter)

1. Rub the trout fillets with a drizzle of olive oil, making sure they're completely coated, and place them under a medium-hot grill, skin side up, with the cherry tomatoes. Cook for 10 minutes until the cherry tomatoes are splitting and the trout skin is crisping.
2. Whizz together the capers, half the parsley, 2 tablespoons of the olive oil and the garlic in a food processor until it forms a coarse paste. Alternatively you can make the paste in a pestle and mortar.
3. Remove the baking tray from under the grill and spread small dollops of the mix over the trout. Scatter the mixed vegetables around the tray.
4. Cook under the grill for a further 5 minutes until the vegetables have warmed through, then serve on a big dish to be shared as it is, or with a watercress salad.

The Rules: Trout is delicious, but as it's a freshwater fish it is very tender. Make sure you don't overcook it under the grill.

The Goodness: Grilled trout contains a staggering 21.5g of protein per 100g and it's packed with beneficial omega-3 oils. It also contains high levels of B12, essential in our bodies for producing blood cells and maintaining a healthy nervous system.

# I HEART PORK AND APRICOT SKEWERS

*Serves 2*
*Prep 10 mins*
*Cook 20 mins*

200g pork fillet
8 apricots (dried or fresh)
olive oil
pinch chilli flakes
pinch salt
100g rocket
2 skewers

1. Cut the pork into large skewer-sized chunks, aiming for 8 chunks per person. Do the same with the apricots.
2. Thread the pork and apricots onto skewers, alternating between the two, drizzle with a little olive oil and sprinkle over the chilli flakes and salt. Cook under a medium-hot grill for 15–20 minutes until the pork is cooked through.
3. Serve with a rocket side salad.

The Rules: This dish is delicious and very simple. Pork tastes great with apricots; make the chunks a similar size so they cook evenly. Check that the pork isn't pink inside but also doesn't become tough and overcooked. These skewers work well on the barbecue too.

The Goodness: Apricots are a great source of vitamin C and also vitamin A, which supports skin and hair health and protects the heart and eyes. They're high in beta-carotene, which helps reduce cholesterol and may help prevent heart disease.

# LEMON AND FENNEL COD

*Serves 2*
*Prep 10 mins*
*Cook 10 mins*

400g cod or 2 cod fillets
olive oil
2 lemons
1 clove garlic, finely sliced
1 white onion, finely sliced
2 fennel bulbs, finely sliced
2 leeks, finely sliced
1 tsp fennel seeds
1 bunch fresh dill, chopped

1. Preheat the oven to 160°C/gas 3.
2. Place the cod on a baking tray, drizzle with olive oil and the juice of half a lemon, season with salt and pepper and bake for 10 minutes, or until cooked through and a little firm to the touch.
3. Heat a splash of olive oil in a pan and sweat down the garlic and onion for 2 minutes before adding the fennel and leeks. Squeeze over the juice of half a lemon, turn the heat down low, then add the fennel seeds and sweat for another 2–4 minutes until the mixture is cooked and slightly wilted.
4. Place half the fennel mix on each plate, then add the cod on top and garnish with fresh lemon slices and dill.

The Rules: This dish works with any good-quality fresh white fish, so you can choose whatever looks good at your fishmongers. Make sure you don't overcook it: check by gently squeezing the fish and carefully sliding a knife into the middle.

The Goodness: Fennel aids digestion, so it's great if you have an upset tum, and it balances your hormones. The aniseed flavour is amazing.

---

## CHOCOLATE AND IRON UP BEEF STEW

*Serves 4*
*Prep 20 mins*
*Cook 1 hour*

olive oil
2 cloves garlic, finely chopped
1 onion, finely chopped
1 green chilli, finely chopped
400g good-quality lean beef steak, chopped
4 tomatoes, chopped
1 tsp curry powder
1 tsp cumin
2 tsp raw cacao powder
2 tsp smoked paprika
juice of 1 lime
100g spinach
½ bunch parsley, chopped

1. Heat a splash of olive oil in a pan and fry the garlic, onion and chilli for 2 minutes. Remove from the pan and set aside.
2. Using the same pan, turn up the heat and fry the beef until golden brown and sealed on all sides.
3. Reduce the heat and return the onion mix to the pan, along with the tomatoes, curry powder, cumin, cacao, paprika, lime

juice, spinach and 150ml water and mix together. Bring to the boil and cook for 2 minutes, then reduce to a medium-low heat. Cover with a lid and cook for 20–30 mins, checking and stirring every 5 minutes.

4. Serve with parsley and a little lime juice sprinkled over the top.

The Rules: This is a perfect dish for sharing and for informal dinner parties. You can prepare it in advance and reheat to serve.

The Goodness: Beef is an excellent source of protein and iron. Iron is a key mineral which helps to deliver oxygen to cells around the body and maintain energy levels.

---

# FILLET STEAK WITH SWEET POTATO WEDGES AND HERBY SAUCE

*Serves 4*
*Prep 10 mins*
*Cook 40 mins*

4 sweet potatoes, cut into wedges
olive oil
1 tsp chilli flakes
1 bunch mint, roughly chopped
1 bunch coriander, roughly chopped
1 fresh chilli, chopped
2 tbsp fish sauce
juice of 1 lime
agave syrup
4 fillet steaks, about 250–300g each

1. Preheat the oven to 180°C/gas 4, putting a baking tray in the oven to heat.
2. Put the sweet potatoes in a bowl, drizzle over a little olive oil, sprinkle over the chilli flakes and season with salt and pepper. Mix it all together, pour into the hot baking tray and cook in the oven for 40 minutes until golden brown, turning every 10 minutes.
3. In a small bowl, mix together the mint, coriander, chilli, fish sauce, lime juice and a splash of agave. Set to one side.
4. When the wedges have about 10 minutes' cooking time left, cook the steaks to your preference under the grill or in a griddle pan, using a very high heat. Leave to rest.
5. Remove the wedges from the oven and divide onto plates with the steak, adding the herby sauce in a small dipping dish on the side before serving.

The Rules: This is really lovely with barbecued steak. Buy the best quality meat you can afford – look for an organic grass-fed variety.

The Goodness: Beef is an excellent source of protein and contains an abundance of iron, a key mineral that carries oxygen to your cells.

# CHINESE FIVE SPICED BEEF ENERGY BOOST

*Serves 4*
*Prep 30 mins*
*Cook 20 mins*

1 tsp Chinese five spice
2 tbsp tamari
2 tbsp apple cider vinegar
3 tbsp black bean sauce
1 thumb-sized piece of ginger, finely chopped
2 red chillies
chilli oil
olive oil
400g beef fillet (or the best cut of beef with no fat you can afford),
    finely sliced
4 spring onions, finely sliced
300g broccoli florets, halved
2 yellow peppers
4 bok choi, cut into chunks
2 tbsp sesame seeds

1.  In a bowl, mix together the Chinese five spice, tamari, vinegar,
    black bean sauce, ginger and 1 finely chopped chilli with a splash
    of chilli oil and pour over the beef. Cover and place in fridge for
    no less than 30 minutes and no more than 2 hours.
2.  Heat a splash of olive oil in a large pan or wok to a high heat.
    Drain off the excess beef marinade into a separate bowl. Cook
    the beef for 2–3 minutes until it browns all over then add all the
    veggies and slowly pour on the rest of the marinade, stirring
    continuously so it doesn't burn. Cook for a further 2–3 minutes.

3. Serve immediately with a scattering of sesame seeds on top and the remaining chilli, cut into slices.

The Rules: Don't overcook the meat: if you can see that the beef is cooked, add the veggies sooner.

The Goodness: Beef is a great source of protein and iron. Iron is in every cell in our bodies; among other things, it helps to carry oxygen from our lungs through our bodies and it supports our muscle function and brain function.

---

## QUINOA, MANGO AND RED ONION SALAD

*Serves 4*
*Prep 10 minutes*
*Cook 15 minutes*

300g quinoa
olive oil
½ pint vegetable stock
2 mangos, finely chopped
1 red onion, finely chopped
½ bunch mint, finely chopped
½ bunch coriander, finely chopped
l lime
pinch red chilli flakes or fresh chilli to taste

1. Rinse the quinoa thoroughly under running water and drain. Heat a splash of olive oil in a pan and add the quinoa and half of the vegetable stock and bring to a simmer. Cook, stirring

regularly, until it thickens, then add splashes of water until the quinoa has sprouted and is fluffy in texture like couscous. Remove from the heat, cover with a lid and let it stand for 5 minutes.

2. Mix together the mangos, red onion, mint and coriander with the juice and zest of the lime.

3. Fold the cooked quinoa into the mango mix, dust with chilli, season with salt and pepper and serve.

The Rules: Get the quinoa to the right consistency: it will keep cooking and fluff up after you remove the pan from the heat, so take it off a couple of minutes before you think it's ready. If you're unsure, keep tasting it. Your palate is the best measure you've got.

The Goodness: High in protein, this dish also has a low GI and is packed with vitamins. It's also rich in carotenoid, which helps protect your skin from the sun. Great on its own or served with fish or white meat.

---

## SKINNY BITCH RED PRAWN AND MANGO CURRY WITH WILD RICE

*Serves 4*
*Prep 15 minutes*
*Cook 30 minutes*

sesame oil
1 spring onion, finely sliced
2 tbsp Thai red curry paste

½ medium butternut squash, finely diced

1 large sweet potato, finely diced

400ml coconut milk

200ml chicken stock

1 tbsp fish sauce

200g fresh or frozen king prawns (partially defrost frozen prawns)

juice of 1 lime

2 fresh mangos, finely diced

400g wild rice

1 bunch coriander, finely chopped

1 red chilli, finely chopped

1. Heat a splash of sesame oil in a deep frying pan over a high heat and fry three-quarters of the spring onion for a few seconds, then add the curry paste and cook for 2 minutes, stirring continuously so it doesn't catch on the bottom.

2. Add the squash and sweet potato cubes to the pan and cook for about 15 minutes.

3. Now add the coconut milk, half the stock and the fish sauce, stir well and simmer for a further 5 minutes.

4. Add the prawns, followed by the lime juice and diced mango and cook for a further 2 minutes, then remove the pan from the heat and allow it to stand for 2 minutes. Check the prawns are cooked through. If I'm using fresh prawns, I normally add them last, after I have removed the pan from the heat.

5. Meanwhile, boil up your wild rice with 1 part rice to 2 parts water and a sprinkle of sea salt. Cook for 5–10 minutes, then cover with a lid and allow to rest for 2 minutes.

6. Serve the curry on top of the rice, sprinkled with the coriander, chilli and remaining spring onion to add texture.

The Rules: Don't bring this dish to the boil, as it's very delicate and boiling will kill the lovely goodness and flavour; a gentle simmer with bubbles arising every couple of seconds is fine.

The Goodness: Prawns are high in protein, omega-3 fatty acids and zinc. Zinc is known to increase levels of leptin, a hormone that regulates the body's energy expenditure, fat storage and appetite. Beware: they are also high in cholesterol, so eating them a few times a week is fine, but don't go crazy with these little pink beauties. Chillies also boost your metabolism so make it as hot as you can take.

# Sweet Treats

## BANANA AND ALMOND LOLLIES

*Serves 1*
*Prep 5 mins*
*Chill 2 hours*

50g almonds
1 banana
coconut milk or coconut yogurt
1 lolly stick

1. Crush your almonds as finely as you can with a rolling pin, making sure there's still some texture, and spread out on a flat saucer or plate.
2. Gently insert the lolly stick halfway into the banana, making sure it doesn't break. Dip the banana into the coconut milk or yogurt, then roll the banana in the almonds, ensuring the whole banana is covered.
3. Place on a baking sheet in the freezer for 2 hours, then it's ready. Put in a plastic tub, these should keep for weeks!

The Rules: Make sure you use big fat bananas; it's tricky to get a lollipop stick into the smaller ones.

The Goodness: Almonds are an amazing food, rich in dietary fibre and vitamin E, which is great for your skin. They're high in natural sugars but very rich in potassium, calcium and magnesium – great for muscles and the nervous system.

# FLOURLESS ALMOND BUTTER CHOCOLATE CHIP BLONDIES

*Serves 16*
*Prep 10 mins*
*Cook 25 mins*

250g natural almond butter
100g manuka honey
1 large egg
¼ tsp salt
½ tsp baking powder
60g dark chocolate chips
pinch chilli flakes

1. Preheat oven to 200°C/gas 6. Grease and line a 20cm square cake tin with baking parchment.
2. In a small bowl, mix together the almond butter, honey, egg, salt and baking powder until well combined, or pop it all into your blender and whizz up until smooth. Then fold in the chocolate chips and mix for another minute.
3. Pour the mix into the tray and bake in the oven for 10–15 minutes until golden.
4. Remove from the oven and leave to cool for 20 minutes.
5. Sprinkle with the chilli flakes. Cut into 16 small squares and serve. These can be frozen and will keep for months or refrigerated for a few days.

The Rules: This is a delicious treat, dense with sweet but healthy ingredients. Maximum 2 pieces a day on treat days only!

The Goodness: Almonds are fantastic for keeping your levels of blood fats healthy, so that you're less likely to get heart disease.

# AVOCADO CHOCOLATE PUDDING

*Serves 2*
*Prep 5 mins*
*Chill 3 hours*

1 orange
2 ripe avocados
2 tbsp raw cacao powder
1 tbsp agave syrup
pinch chilli powder
splash vanilla extract
pinch salt
fresh blueberries and mint, for garnish

1. Zest and juice the orange. Place all the ingredients except for the blueberries and mint into food processor and blitz until you end up with a mousse-like consistency. Alternatively, you can mash the ingredients together and stir until they're as smooth as you can get them.
2. Place into small glasses and refrigerate for at least 3 hours. (The pudding can be prepared a day in advance.)
3. Garnish with fresh blueberries and mint before serving.

The Rules: Avocados are high in fat (around 14g per fruit), so enjoy them occasionally. This isn't a pud to make every day.

The Goodness: Avocado is a superfood, rich in protein, 'happy' fats and vitamin E. It's actually a fruit, but it's great used in savoury cooking and salads.

# THE ULTIMATE CRUMBLE

*Serves 6*
*Prep 10 mins*
*Cook 30 mins*

4 peaches
8 apricots
5 tbsp maple syrup or dark agave syrup
a splash of vanilla extract with seeds
1 lemon
50g ground almonds
50g macadamia nuts
50g pecan nuts
30g pumpkin seeds
4 Medjool dates
10g goji berries
pinch cinnamon
pinch nutmeg
pinch salt
80g quinoa flakes
10g flaked almonds

1. Preheat the oven to 200°C/gas 6.
2. Stone the fruit, chop into segments and put in a fairly deep baking tray. Pour over 3 tablespoons of the maple or agave syrup, add a splash of vanilla extract and the zest and juice of the lemon, and mix together. Roast in oven for 10–15 minutes.
3. For the crumble, chuck all the nuts (except the flaked almonds), seeds, dates, goji berries, cinnamon, nutmeg and salt into a blender and whizz up until crumbly but still a bit coarse, to give

it texture. If you don't have a blender, roll your sleeves up and get chopping!

4. Add the quinoa flakes and the remaining 2 tablespoons of syrup to the mix and whizz for a few seconds to blend it all together.
5. Sprinkle the crumble mix over the fruits in the baking tray, scatter the flaked almonds over the top and bake for 20–25 minutes.

The Rules: This is another sweet treat and tastes delicious. It's packed with goodness but shouldn't be eaten more than once or twice a week.

The Goodness: Almonds are the champions of fat-shedding nuts as they help regulate blood sugar and lower cholesterol, and not all the calories in them are absorbed. Apricots are packed with vitamin A to support your skin. You'll feel younger and healthier after one bowlful.

---

# FOREVER YOUNG VANILLA ROASTED PEACHES

*Serves 4*
*Prep 5 mins*
*Cook 30 mins*

coconut oil
8 ripe peaches
1 vanilla pod, split in half
2 tsp vanilla extract with seeds
agave syrup
1 orange

pinch cinnamon
pinch nutmeg

1. Preheat the oven to 200°C/gas 6. Put a splash of coconut oil in a roasting tray and place in the oven.
2. Halve and stone the peaches and place them in a bowl. Add the vanilla pod, vanilla extract, agave and the zest and juice of the orange to the peaches, mix it all together and allow to infuse for 5 minutes.
3. Place the peaches face down in the baking tray, which should be hot enough for the oil to sizzle, setting aside any excess juice. Roast for 10 minutes. Check that they are well roasted and then turn them over. Sprinkle the excess juice and the cinnamon and nutmeg over the top and roast for a further 10 minutes.
4. Serve on a plate with a trickle of the roasting juices over the top and an extra dusting of cinnamon.

The Rules: Another delicious treat that's also dense with sweet but healthy ingredients. It's fine to enjoy in moderation – once or twice a week is perfect.

The Goodness: Packed with vitamins including skin-friendly vitamin A, peaches are a good healthy source of fibre, passing very quickly through your digestive system.

# MOOD-LIFTING BBQ FRUIT KEBABS AND DIPPING CHOCOLATE

*Serves 4*
*Prep 20 mins*
*Cook 10 mins*

1 pineapple
1 small punnet strawberries
4 kiwi fruit
2 peaches
juice of 1 lemon
100g desiccated coconut
200g dark chocolate (70% cocoa solids)
2 tbsp coconut oil
8 bamboo skewers

1. Cut all the fruit into 2.5cm chunks and thread onto the skewers, making sure the fruit combos are varied, for example one chunk of pineapple, strawberry, peach and kiwi, then repeat.
2. Squeeze lemon juice over the skewered fruit and then roll in a plate of desiccated coconut until lightly covered.
3. Place the kebabs on a hot barbecue or griddle pan or pop under the grill for 10 minutes until the coconut is turning golden brown.
4. Over a bain-marie (a pan of boiling water with a bowl on top), melt the chocolate and mix in the coconut oil. Place in a dipping bowl with the skewers on the side and serve.

The Rules: This lovely light dessert or snack is a real fresh treat and easy to prepare; it also looks lovely with the different colours. It's best when cooked on a barbecue for a smoky but fruity taste. This dish is high in natural sugars, so it's not a treat for every day.

The Goodness: Fruit is packed with nutritious properties and the healthy chemicals in dark chocolate help keep the arteries elastic. Dark chocolate can also protect your skin and improve your mood as it contains PEA (phenylethylamine), a natural mood enhancer.

---

## CHOC 'O' NUTS – THE AMAZING SNACK BAR

*Serves 4*
*Prep 15 mins*
*Chill 5 hours*

100g almonds
100g cashew nuts
50g pumpkin seeds
200g Medjool dates
100g almond butter
4 tbsp maple syrup
50g desiccated coconut
2 tsp vanilla extract with seeds
300g dark chocolate chips (70% cocoa solids)
1 tbsp coconut oil

1. Blend the almonds, cashews and pumpkin seeds in a food processor until finely ground. Add the dates, almond butter, maple syrup, desiccated coconut and vanilla extract and blend until it's all sticky and mixed.
2. Line a medium-sized baking tray about 20cm square and 5cm deep with baking parchment. Press the nutty mix into the tray and place in the fridge to set.

3. Melt the chocolate in a bain-marie (a pan of boiling water with a bowl on top) and stir in the coconut oil, then remove from the heat.

4. Remove the nutty mix from the fridge and pour the melted chocolate over the top, spread it out into an even layer. If you want to use less chocolate, dip a spoon into the melted mix and trickle it over the nut mixture to create chocolate lines on your bars.

5. Return to the fridge and leave to set for 5–10 hours, or overnight if possible.

6. Cut into rectangles about 5cm x 2.5cm to serve, or use a shaped biscuit cutter to make the bars more fun. These will last for a week in an airtight container.

The Rules: This is a sweet treat and while it contains a lot of energy and heath-protecting ingredients, it should only be eaten twice a week maximum.

The Goodness: These ingredients deliver an awesome energy boost as well as supporting your brain function. The bars are also very filling and contains lots of good fats and protein. Chocolate is a known mood enhancer and has powerful antioxidant properties.

# Foods That Can Go Five Ways

Here are some dead easy meals with different ingredients that can be swapped in and out.

## MIXED GREEN SALAD WITH PESTO-PACKED PROTEIN

*Serves 1*
*Prep 5 mins*
*Cook 5–15 mins*

100g bag mixed leaves
pesto sauce (buy readymade in a jar)

*plus one of the following*
1 chicken breast, grilled
1 285g steak, grilled
1 salmon fillet, grilled
1 avocado, sliced
2 eggs (poached, hard-boiled or scrambled)

Add your choice of meat, fish, avocado or eggs to the mixed leaves, drizzle over 1 teaspoon of pesto and mix together. Try to change the protein source on alternate days. This is a great option for lunch: you'll get the protein and carbs you need and stay full for the day.

# MIXED MEDITERRANEAN VEG WITH EXTRA VIRGIN OLIVE OIL AND SEA SALT

*Serves 1*
*Prep 5 mins*
*Cook 20 mins*

1 tomato
1 courgette
1 red onion
1 red pepper
olive oil
salt to taste

*plus one of the following (you get an extra two options with this*
*one!)*
1 chicken breast, grilled
1 285g steak, grilled
2 lamb chops, grilled
2 pork chops, grilled
1 fillet of salmon (or tuna or any other fave fishy), grilled
1 avocado, sliced
2 eggs, hard-boiled

Preheat oven to 200°C/gas 6. Cut the veg into similar-sized chunks, place in a baking tray or dish, drizzle with a little olive oil, season with a little salt to taste and roast for 20 minutes. Then serve with your choice of meat, fish, avocado or eggs. This is a good option for dinner, as you will probably have more time in the evening to cook.

# MASHED CHILLI AND GARLIC SWEET POTATO WITH WILTED SPINACH

*Serves 1*
*Prep 5 mins*
*Cook 20 mins*

1 large sweet potato, peeled and cubed
olive oil
½ clove garlic, finely chopped
½ red chilli, finely chopped
½ bunch coriander, chopped
100g spinach

*plus one of the following*
1 pork chop, grilled
2 lamb chops, grilled
1 salmon fillet, grilled
1 sea bass, mackerel or another delicious white fish, grilled
6 king prawns, grilled

Boil the sweet potato until it is cooked, then drain. Mash with the olive oil, then mix in the garlic, chilli and coriander. Wilt the spinach in two teaspoons of boiling water and serve with the sweet-potato mash and your choice of meat or fish. This dish is a great support for your sight and energy levels.

# RATATOUILLE

*Serves 2*
*Prep 10 mins*
*Cook 20 mins*

olive oil
1 clove garlic, finely chopped
1 red chilli, finely chopped
1 red onion, chopped
1 aubergine
1 red pepper
1 courgette
2 beef tomatoes
1 tin passata

*plus one of the following*
1 chicken breast, grilled or steamed
1 285g steak, grilled
1 chicken thigh, grilled
1 tuna steak, grilled
1 white fish fillet, grilled

Heat a splash of olive oil in a pan and sweat off the garlic, chilli and onion for 2 minutes. Chop the other veg into pieces about 2.5cm in size and chuck into the pan. Add the passata and cook for 15–20 minutes until everything is tender and the sauce is reduced. Serve with your choice of meat or fish. This dish is fab – the rich tomato sauce gives your body a boost to help fight cancerous cells.

# SUPER-SPEEDY STIR FRY

*Serves 2*
*Prep 5 mins*
*Cook 5 mins*

coconut oil or sesame seed oil
1 clove garlic, finely chopped
1 red chilli, finely chopped
1 thumb-sized piece ginger, peeled and finely chopped
1 red pepper, sliced
1 green pepper, sliced
1 yellow pepper, sliced
1 white onion, sliced
1 small head broccoli, cut into florets
100g spinach
2 tbsp tamari

*plus one of the following*
2 chicken breasts, sliced
12 raw king prawns
350g pork fillet, sliced
350g good-quality steak, sliced
350g turkey breast, sliced

Heat a splash of oil in a wok and fry the finely chopped garlic, chilli and ginger for 20 seconds. Then add your choice of meat or fish and fry at high heat for 2 minutes. Add the peppers, onion and broccoli, then last of all the spinach and tamari, and fry fast for about 2 minutes. Make sure the veg stay crunchy and the meat is cooked to your liking. Serve immediately. This dish gives you a great nutrient lift as the veggies should still be slightly raw, retaining their crunch.

# NINE

# How to Stay Motivated – Beating the Cravings and Sugar Withdrawal

Now you've got started, how do you stay on the straight and narrow? It's all too easy to slip back into bad habits. Falling off the wagon is as inevitable as a DNA test during an episode of *Jeremy Kyle*. I still do it sometimes and so does every other dieter I know – or at least the ones honest enough to admit it. On a night out with the girls last year, I ate a kebab at 3 a.m., and that was after an early-evening three-course dinner and some dancing. I'd drunk far too many vodka and Red Bulls and was hungover the next day despite my doner, so I followed up in the morning with a bacon sandwich, a white bagel and a full-fat latte, all before 10 a.m. – if I fall off the wagon, I do it in style. I won't go into detail about what it did to my insides; but I do know, with hindsight, that I let it affect my mindset for far too long.

Falling off the wagon is a fact of dieting. You're going to do it at some point, if you haven't already, and that's fine – but what's far from fine is using it as an excuse to ditch the whole thing and go back to your old ways. Everyone makes mistakes – like when I was sixteen and a size 16 and thought a boob tube would suit me.

But we learn from them and don't keep making the same ones. If and when you fall off the wagon, enjoy it, indulge yourself, accept you've made a mistake, then pull yourself up by the bootstraps and carry on. Don't keep thinking you've let yourself down and wasted all the hard work you've put in – you haven't. If and when it happens, see it for what it is: a temporary lapse in judgement. Don't keep beating yourself over the head with it or you really will derail every-thing you've been working towards. Instead, try some of these tricks to help you stay focused on your goals.

## TARGETS AND REWARDS

When I realized there was no substitute for eating less and moving more, I got my head down and set myself some targets and rewards. You see, I knew I wanted to end up under 10 stone and a size 10, but waiting until I lost 6 stone to celebrate made me feel like I was looking at a prison sentence. I decided to mark every stone I lost with a treat. Mini-milestones and rewards will always make a diet easier to stick to.

In terms of treats, it's OK to draw up a list of your favourite 'old' foods and put them (firmly) in the 'milestone treat' category. But make sure you mix these up with some non-food rewards, like a massage or manicure or a new pair of shoes. In the long run, most nutritionists reckon that continuing to use foods as rewards will only keep that emotional connection with foods going. And demonizing some foods as 'naughty' means you'll just crave them even more. A bit like when your mum told you not to do something when you were a kid – it was always the thing you'd turn around and do straight away. So celebrate every time you lose half a stone or every time you lose an inch, but don't always make the celebration food related. Treat yourself to that bag you've been hankering after or buy the killer heels you know you'll rarely wear. For me though, treat *numero uno* was a dark-chocolate fountain, and with 84lb to lose, I set my first milestone at 14lb.

# Sugar Withdrawal

It took me over a month to shift that first stone. While the pounds fell off pretty fast and consistently, I was suffering with mood swings and insomnia which I couldn't get rid of. My skin was a mess and I was shaky and snappy – imagine being premenstrual constantly and you'll get the picture. I put it down to changing my lifestyle and the stress of putting my body through physical exercise for the first time ever. But the grogginess and slight feeling of constant nausea wouldn't shift.

Being the hypochondriac I am, I started trawling the internet looking up my symptoms. I was convinced I had something that would derail my dream of being a size 10 before I even got started, but within a few clicks I realized I was coming down from a sugar addiction I'd been feeding for the last twenty-five years. I'd have unbearable stomach cramps, worse than my lactose-intolerance ones, which left me unable to train, and I'd either be constipated for weeks or have bowels so loose you'd think I'd just been called into the *Big Brother* house for the first time. But worst of all, I started craving sugar like a junkie craves a fix. Tea and coffee were completely unpalatable without it and I'd feel myself getting turned on by the confectionery counter in the petrol station. If I so much as caught Lukey with a Crunchie wrapper in his pocket, I'd fly off the handle at him, accusing him of bringing sweets into the house to tempt me and derail my diet. I became completely unpredictable and my mood swings were difficult even for me to cope with.

You see, the white stuff is far more addictive than the brown stuff. Imagine being a heroin addict and seeing it on sale everywhere, from corner shops to petrol forecourts to vending machines. Suddenly I couldn't step out the house without seeing an advert on the side of a bus for a new Cadbury's bar or watching someone in the car at traffic lights devouring a milkshake. I'd watch people in the park drinking their full-fat Cokes while I was doing reps and sets like a woman possessed. I was trying desperately hard to beat my addiction, but temptation was literally everywhere.

But recognizing and admitting to my addiction was only the start of what is an ongoing battle that will probably continue for the rest of my life. There's no Priory for sugar addicts, no Twelve Step programme, no sponsors to support us. A third of all primary-school leavers are obese or overweight, but there's big business in this legal drug, so the incentive to fight it and protect the next generation from ending up like me isn't a priority.

There are few statistics on sugar addiction because only a small number of doctors, physicians and professors have done enough research for it to be recognized as a condition. There are other factors at play for obesity and diabetes diagnoses, but a lot of our weight issues stem from sugar addiction. How many people do you know who get by every day at work on cans of Coke? Or can't resist that biscuit in the afternoon? They're all potential signs of an addiction to sugar, and you don't have to be a size 20 to be a sugar addict.

Going cold turkey to rid myself of my addiction is one of the hardest things I've ever had to do in my life. I'd come back from the gym exhausted and sit and cry. Sobbing my heart out, longing for one final Yorkie or a last glug of Ribena. You see, for me, sugar and love were inextricably linked. From my dad weaning me on rice pudding to my nan and I devouring cream cakes and Chelsea buns at motorway service stations, sharing sweet treats with friends and family was a way of showing them you loved them and were loved in return.

I was trying hard to beat my addiction and lose weight at the same time. Both were just as difficult, but the morning I stepped onto the scales and saw that I had lost my first stone, I honestly think I was more excited about the prospect of the chocolate fountain than the number between my feet. My heart was pounding with excitement when I called Luke and told him tonight was his lucky night – I'd banned sugar from the house completely after being tempted to commit GBH to get my hands on his biscuit Boost. So the poor bugger was the same as me: far more excited about the prospect of sugar passing his lips than he was about his fiancé losing her first 14lb.

We were both euphoric when I got home that night. I'd bought some Veuve Clicquot, something else I hadn't had for over a month, he'd got fresh strawberries from Marks and the chocolate fountain was heating up. We were both excited and randy and within minutes the first glass of fizz went to my head. I hadn't drunk for five weeks, and was feeling giddy when I took my first bright-red shiny fruit and parted the velvety waterfall of dark silky chocolate with it. I twisted it around until all I could see was a hint of red by the deep-green stalk and then devoured it in a second. Dark chocolate dripped down my chin as I bit through to the tender, sweet, fragrant strawberry underneath, the two flavours melding into one sweet crescendo of sugar. I drained my glass of fizz to cleanse my palate for the next one while holding Lukey's gaze. If there's one thing this former size 20 randy mare knows how to do, it's how to eat in a provocative manner.

But my plans of ravaging the box of strawberries and then my Luke went awry within minutes of eating my first strawb. Having not eaten so much as a grain of sugar for weeks, my tum was gurgling loud enough to ruin any hint of a romantic mood. I hadn't factored in that my longed-for treat might make me ill. Within twenty minutes sitting down for my treat, I was stuck on the toilet and spent the rest of the night there. It was like I'd overdosed on laxatives. The chocolate and fizz were far too rich for a sugar addict who'd been battling to stay clean for over a month. Putting that much sweet stuff into my body in one go gave me a mini-overdose. Luke kept checking on me to see if I still fancied a bit of hanky-panky, but three hours later I climbed into bed and kissed my sleeping prince on the cheek before falling into a spent, exhausted sleep.

It turns out every cloud really does have a silver lining, though: when I got on the scales the next morning, I'd lost another three pounds in addition to the first stone. But while I was delighted and waxed lyrical to Luke about how that many hours spent on the bog had been worth it in a way, I couldn't help but sense he'd have been happier with a bit of nooky.

Not surprisingly, I swore off the white stuff again.

# How to Control Your Cravings

There are plenty of things I've craved over the years, from Irn-Bru bars and penny chews bought with my pop's sweetie fund when I was a kid to chip butties, spring rolls and sweet-and-sour chicken balls with egg fried rice in my teens. Not to mention dark-chocolate fountains with fruit in my twenties.

Before I'd given into my cravings whether I was trying to lose weight or not, which always led to a lot of self-loathing and misery.

Whether I longed for freshly baked bread from the supermarket with plenty of cold salty butter melting into it or a Sara Lee lemon meringue pie fresh from the oven with extra sugar and cream on top, I'd try to ignore it or sate the feelings with something else, but a craving is irrational and can strike at any time.

Even now, just the other morning, when I'd had poached eggs and smoked salmon for breakfast. Why was I craving sweet milky tea with a custard cream half an hour later? Cravings are one of the biggest derailers of diets. Sticking to a healthy eating plan would be a cinch were it not for the fact we all end up craving something we shouldn't eat. Don't get me wrong, I love sushi – but sometimes I find myself craving a big Fray Bentos steak and kidney pie with lashings of buttery mashed potato, like I used to eat when I was a child.

Can you imagine how much easier it'd be to stick to a diet and lose weight if we weren't troubled by food cravings? If we didn't 'miss' the old foods we'd given up? And why is it that the foods that we absolutely, definitely have to eat this second are chocolate, chips or warm bread with lashings of butter, rather than a healthy bowl of fruit salad?

Firstly, food cravings tend to be for high-fat or sugary foods quite simply because they taste good and bring immediate gratification to the chemical receptors in our brains. This is why we crave 'naughty' foods rather than 'good' foods like celery.

Secondly, food cravings are more likely to strike when hunger gets the best of us, which can occur due to skipping meals, poor meal planning or not having suitable snacks to hand. Studies have shown that we tend to make poor nutritional choices when hunger strikes because we're led by the grumbling in our bellies, rather than by the contents of the fridge. But not all cravings are created equal. In fact, worryingly, less than 40 per cent of cravers reported being hungry when they experienced cravings. A craving is something stronger than hunger and the two things are not always linked.

One thing for sure is that cravings are very common. A study of over a thousand people published in the *International Journal of Eating Disorders* found that 28 per cent of women and 13 per cent of men had experienced a strong urge to eat specific foods more than once a week during the past 6 months.

But the kicker is we're far more likely to crave foods that we think of as 'naughty', foods we've been taught are bad since childhood, than we are to crave something that's healthy and good for us. In Britain, our favourite craved foods include chocolate, cakes, crisps and chips, which may be a reflection of the type of foods we were given as treats when we were young, things that have come to be associated with comfort. Chocolate in particular is an intensely desirable food because of the way it melts at close to body temperature, giving that sensuous feeling in your mouth.

But while cravings are linked to pleasure centres in the brain and can be activated just by seeing a food, they're also linked to hormones. Ever wondered why you can finish a box of Celebrations a couple of days before your period? When asked, 60 per cent of American women and 34 per cent of Spanish women said they specifically crave chocolate just before a period, which indicates a strong hormonal basis for cravings.

Some scientists have also suggested that food cravings may be expressions of wisdom on the part of our bodies, which are telling us to eat particular foods in order to get the nutrients we are missing. If we craved red meat in caveman times it would probably have been because we needed more protein in our bodies, but these days we question our cravings because of the abundance of foods available to us. There's actually no strong evidence that food cravings are linked to nutritional deficiency. If there were, your go-to food for a magnesium deficiency would be okra, not chocolate.

The most likely cause of food cravings, particularly those that we give in to and that can lead to bingeing, is our emotions, particularly feeling fed up, bored or sad. Cravings and comfort eating aren't so far apart. They're both negative, unnecessary and can derail even the most determined dieter. Comfort eating and giving into cravings delivers a temporary solution to unhappiness because they raise your blood-sugar levels and increase the amount of feel-good chemicals produced by the brain. But uncontrolled eating can actually make us feel worse, because as the number on the scales increases, we begin to loathe ourselves for not having more self-control.

## BEAT THE CRAVINGS

Cravings and comfort eating are a natural part of your journey. But there are ways you can beat them and reduce the number of times you give into temptation.

### Hang on in there

If you're craving food but you're not hungry, the urge will pass. Set a timer for twenty minutes, or longer if you think you can stand it. If you are still genuinely hungry after the time has elapsed, go ahead and eat. The fact that you waited rather than indulging instantly is something to be proud of.

### Have healthy snacks to hand

If you prevent your blood sugar dipping, you'll find you won't desire a sugar hit as much. Keep nuts and seeds in the cupboard, crudités in the fridge, fruit in the fruit bowl and always make sure you have something to hand in your bag when you're out so you don't give in to the Co-op confectionery counter.

### Try drinking a glass of water or cup of tea instead

Drinking liquids can fill your stomach and take the edge off your desire to eat. Take your time and really taste your drink. Distracting your mouth with either a hot or cold drink may go some way to helping you forget you were craving a biccie.

### Snack on some protein

A handful of prawns or half a can of tuna may also break the grip of a sugar craving when you are in imminent danger of overdosing on sweets. A dose of protein will make you feel full almost instantly.

### Make your surroundings less food 'toxic'

This could mean clearing your cupboard of chocolate, always taking a packed lunch with you so you don't succumb to fast food at lunchtime, or walking a different way to the shops so you don't pass the bakery.

### Buy individual, not family-sized, packs of the foods you're most likely to crave

No one will notice if one Kit Kat out of a pack of fourteen goes missing, but you might get found out if you've eaten the last one left in the cupboard – that knowledge might just be enough to dissuade you from eating it.

### Break any habits that bring on cravings

If you're used to having a cuppa and a biscuit after *This Morning* every day, paint your nails instead or make sure you switch to a different channel before the titles roll. Cravings can often be associated with routine, so try to switch yours up.

### Chew gum

You can usually stall a craving for something sweet by chewing a stick of sugar-free gum. It will go some way to satisfy your lust for something unhealthy, and more importantly it will keep your mouth busy for a while – hopefully long enough for the craving to pass.

### Add feelings into your food diary

Write down everything you eat and how you were feeling when you ate it. It will help you to identify when your cravings strike and to be aware of the emotions driving them. You'll soon be able to establish which emotion usually kick-starts your cravings, be it boredom, stress, anxiety or loneliness, and then you can tackle the emotion and not just the craving.

### Get some sleep

Not getting enough shut-eye is linked with weight-gain, probably because your body craves sugars in an attempt to overcome tiredness and stay awake.

### Eat a high-protein lunch to keep you fuller

Protein is the most satiating of all nutrients. Choose a protein-packed lunch and the chances are you'll find it easier to curb a 4 p.m. sugar craving.

So we all know what cravings are and why they may strike. But what do they mean? Why did I constantly crave chocolate when my mate Jeanette always craved crisps? Some schools of thought suggest that the sensations created by the foods we crave can go some way to explaining *why* we crave *what* we do, *when* we do.

### Crunchy

Craving crunchy foods can mean you're suffering from stress and dealing with a lot of tension. Crunching your jaws up and down can relieve pressure – the oral equivalent of going a few rounds with the punch bag in the gym.

### Creamy

Creamy foods, especially milk, cream and cheese, contain a chemical that helps relieve anxiety and insecurity. If you're constantly reaching for the Ben & Jerry's, could that be at the heart of your craving?

### Chewy

If you particularly crave chewy flapjacks or something else you have to masticate for a while, you could be suffering with underlying feelings of tension. Chewing slowly releases tension; just ask Sir Alex Ferguson – in twenty-five years as manager of Manchester United, he was never seen on the touchline without his Wrigley's.

### Spicy

Craving spicy foods can signal boredom with your existence. Heat and chillies awaken our taste buds and digestive systems; you may be transferring to your palate the need to wake up your life.

In addition to specific textures, some small-scale studies have claimed that foods we crave can tell us plenty about our emotional state in general. Here are some examples.

## CHOCOLATE

Cocoa butter melts sensuously in the mouth. It also symbolizes love and gratitude, reinforcing on a psychological level its position as our number one food fantasy. According to research, it accounts for about half of all craving episodes. Chocolate contains phenylethylamine, the chemical naturally produced in the brain when we experience a romantic love, which may explain why we reach for the Galaxy after a break-up!

### How to control it

Anecdotally, women who increase their intake of the mineral magnesium by taking a supplement, or by eating nuts, whole grains and spinach, reduce hormonally-driven chocolate cravings. Another way to fight a craving is to only eat chocolate when you're full. Researchers at University College London found that subjects told to eat chocolate when they weren't hungry found their cravings became weaker, while eating it on an empty stomach made their cravings stronger.

## STEAK

If you're craving meat, you're probably properly hungry, rather than just seeking emotional satisfaction. Despite lots of theories floating around, there's no evidence that craving meat means you're protein or iron deficient.

### How to control it

Make sure you're eating enough high-quality protein, but don't have red meat every day (too much red and processed meat is linked with colon cancer) and keep your portion sizes reasonable – ideally no bigger than a pack of cards.

## MARMITE AND OTHER SALTY FOODS

A study at the University of Haifa in Israel found that people whose mothers had experienced bad morning sickness were the most likely to crave salty foods, perhaps because of pre-birth exposure to loss of fluids and sodium. Craving Marmite, Worcester sauce or parmesan cheese could also mean you're hooked on the so-called fifth taste, umami – a satisfying savoury taste sensation produced by glutamic acid. Sometimes a strong salt craving can be a sign of an adrenal gland problem.

### How to control it

Satisfy your craving with foods that contain salt only on the outside – like salted peanuts – which can be less salty overall than soup and cereals in which salt permeates the whole food. Dried porcini mushrooms are a great way to satisfy a taste for umami flavours without a dose of blood-pressure-raising salt. If your salt craving is newly developed and strong, see your GP.

## JELLY BEANS

Your yen could also be for marshmallows or wine gums, but whichever your fix, you're craving the instant lift that sugar gives to your energy level. These cravings can be self-perpetuating, as a rapid rise in your blood glucose is followed by a rapid fall, stimulating a further round of craving for sweets.

### How to control it

Never skip meals, and avoid processed carbohydrates that are digested quickly and cause your blood-sugar to fluctuate. A high-protein snack (chicken pieces or a scrambled egg) may also break the grip of a sugar craving when you are in imminent danger of overdosing on sweets.

## DONUTS

Cakes, biscuits, donuts and ice-cream combine sugar and fat in the most compelling way, possibly because we're genetically predisposed to search out both. In evolutionary terms, sweetness indicates a food is not poisonous, whereas fat, because of its high calorie count, represents the most efficient way to prevent starvation.

### How to control it

Try to meet the inbuilt need for sweetness and fat by eating moderate portions of healthier sweet or oily foods, such as dried fruit, nuts and avocados.

Another way to tackle your cravings is to try to establish at which stage of hunger you're used to eating. How often do we think about how hungry we actually are before food?

I used to eat within half an hour of waking up in the morning, usually with a bit of a hangover. I'd snack mid-morning or graze for a couple of hours and then have lunch between 12 noon and 1 p.m. Then I'd have dinner between 5 p.m. and 7 p.m., followed by a snack or two and some more grazing in front of the telly between 9 p.m. and midnight. Just how hungry was I each and every time I shoved food in my mouth? Not very, if memory serves correctly. I ate out of habit, because the hands on the clock dictated that I should. How many of us actually ask ourselves about our hunger levels before we open the fridge door or the bread bin? We're used to eating by the clock and so whether or not we're actually hungry rarely comes into the equation.

If you concentrate on hunger, you'll start to get more in tune with your system and your hunger cycles, and that can only be a good thing. Regularly rating your hunger on a scale of one to ten throughout the day will help you to establish when you're at your weakest or hungriest or most bored – and therefore more prone to cravings.

Start with a scale of one to ten. One is ravenously, stomach growlingly, eat-the-postman-when-he-delivers-the-mail hungry, whereas ten is completely stuffed. As the ideal is for you to feel reasonably hungry before a meal and comfortably satisfied afterwards, you should be aiming not to start eating until you register a four or below on the scale, and you should stop putting food in your mouth when you hit seven or eight.

If you find yourself constantly sitting at either end of the scale, you're damaging your system, your metabolism and your chances of losing weight. Don't wait until you're ravenous before you start eating, and make sure you stop eating before you're full. Your brain takes fifteen minutes to catch up with your body when you're eating, so if you stop eating when you feel full, you'll feel full to the point of queasiness in fifteen minutes' time. Stop eating when you feel almost full, and then when your brain catches up with your belly you'll feel sated and happy, rather than like Santa after Christmas dinner.

The chances are that if you're heading for your dinner plate when you're ravenous, you'll be swallowing your food before you've even properly chewed it. Chewing helps break down the enzymes in food we need for digestion, so if you're swallowing your meals without chewing properly, there's every chance you're denying your body some vital nutrients from what you're eating. Chewing thoroughly before swallowing, putting your knife and fork down between bites and taking at least twenty minutes to eat a meal are all great tips to help you slow down, and notice and appreciate, what you are eating. It's a way to naturally self-regulate your intake of food, and you'll find you taste it more too.

Cravings are often stimulated by our brains: we don't need that Bounty bar nutritionally, but our brain wants it and can create a false 'head hunger' to try to convince us we're actually famished. Stomach hunger is real hunger. But how do you differentiate between the two?

### Head hunger

This is something you're likely to experience in association with negative emotions like frustration or anger, or as a response to stress, boredom or habit. Do you find yourself reaching for the Werther's during a meeting at work? Or finishing a bowl of popcorn in front of the latest episode of *Luther*? You don't actually need to eat – you're responding to head hunger.

Do you find yourself craving a bowl of Frosties after seeing Tony the Tiger jumping off the high diving board in the TV ad? You've fallen prey to non-hungry eating stimulated by the food adverts on TV.

Head hunger is like a nagging voice in your head that convinces you that, as you're having a bad day, it's fine to crack open the kids' cookies and polish off seven in one sitting.

### Stomach hunger

This is more of a physical sensation, when your stomach feels rumbly and empty. But if your tum is actually growling, you've let yourself get too low on the hunger scale. Our food choices tend to deteriorate the stronger hunger becomes, so that when we pop to the sandwich shop for lunch, we're more likely to grab the stodgy wrap rather than wait for the salad to be made up fresh for us.

Stomach hunger increases in intensity the longer we try to ignore it. If you fancy a packet of crisps and distract yourself for twenty minutes only to find you still want it, you're hungry. But before you scoff the Salt 'n' Shake, try eating something better instead, like a banana, then give yourself another twenty minutes and if you still want your fried potatoes, go ahead.

If your tum is rumbling despite the fact that you ate a couple of hours ago, turn your thoughts to *what* you ate. If it was nutritionally poor, your stomach and brain will still require nutrients, despite the volume of whatever you've eaten. Generally we shouldn't be plagued by hunger pangs and stomach rumbles until at least three or four hours after a meal. If you're feeling hungry sooner than that, the chances are your meals aren't nutritionally balanced and don't contain enough nutrients for your body to function.

There'll be a lot of times when you may feel like falling off the wagon, but giving in to cravings can be the deadliest of diet sins. Your trainer or gym buddy will notice if you miss a workout and your bloke will notice if you've suddenly stuffed the fridge full of crap; but cravings, like any addiction, are still there with you in the middle of the night. They're in your head, and that's where you have to do battle with them. And as anyone who's tried to overcome an addiction knows, the demons in your head can be the hardest ones to beat. But when you do, the victory is that bit sweeter.

# What to Do When You Want a Takeaway

My treat day isn't always a Sunday: sometimes (with Lukey's persuasion) I get a takeaway on a Friday or Saturday night instead. He knows I don't need too much persuading. So while he tees up the movie for the night, I have a rummage through our drawer of takeaway menus. But all takeaways are not created equal. You can choose something super stodgy, or you can be good – indulge yourself but not too much. And to save you putting in all the hard work I did to research the subject, here are the healthiest takeaway meals you can order.

## INDIAN

Two of the best:
- Tandoori chicken
- Chicken tikka

The healthiest Indian dish is a sauce-free one, such as tandoori or tikka. Alternatively, you could choose any starter you like and bulk it out with salad, dhal and a poppadom so that it still feels like you're getting a good meal. A non-creamy vegetable curry can be a good bet too.

*Top tips*
- Choose just one accompanying carb: rice or naan, for example, not both.
- Only eat half your main dish – the portions are usually gigantic.

- Leave some sauce behind – most curries are swimming in it and it's the most fattening bit.

## CHINESE

Two of the best:
- Szechuan prawns and vegetables
- Chicken in black bean sauce

Steamed or stir-fry dishes that don't have any battered bits (or crispy anywhere in the title) are the best choices. But don't eat too much rice – half a portion of boiled rice is more than ample, honest! If you've nobody to share with, bin half before tucking in to avoid being tempted.

*Top tips*
- Avoid fattening sides like spring rolls, crispy seaweed and prawn crackers.
- Try a portion of stir-fried vegetable as a lighter alternative to rice.
- Ask for your meal to be cooked without MSG (the better Chinese restaurants shouldn't use it anyway). It makes even average-tasting food moreish and harder to resist.

## TURKISH

Two of the best:
- Chicken shish kebab with salad and pitta
- Falafel, salad and hummus

For a healthier option than the classic doner, go for a shish kebab – a skewer of whole cuts of meat, usually grilled. Alternatively, keep things more slimline with falafel and hummus – they're high in carbs but not the fat-releasing carbs that do the most damage.

*Top tips*

- Step away from the doner: trading standards officers have found some doners containing up to 22 per cent fat and up to 12g of fluid-retaining salt – that's two heaped teaspoons, double the recommended daily intake.
- Watch your sauces: chilli is the best of a bad lot.
- Ask for it without pitta and your thighs will thank you.

## THAI

Two of the best:

- Gai pad med ma-muang (chicken with cashew nuts)
- Moo pad king (pork fried with ginger)

These quick stir-fried dishes aren't weighed down with oil or creamy sauces. Ginger helps to cut through any digestive discomfort, and pork and chicken are good low-fat sources of protein.

*Top tips*

- Ditch the sides and go for hot and sour Thai soup as a starter instead – it'll fill you up.

## MEXICAN

Two of the best:

- Vegetarian chilli quesadilla (without cheese)
- Steak and pepper fajita (easy on the sour cream, heavier on the salsa)

Cheese-free and preferably in a spinach tortilla, a veggie chilli quesadilla counts as one of your five a day and the beans in the chilli keep your energy up without too much waistline damage. Steak fajitas can also be a balanced main, containing vitamin C and iron to protect against anaemia.

*Top tips*

- Better to have one less carb-rich wrap or taco and a bit more veg, bean and protein filling.
- Nachos are so difficult when it comes to portion control and slip down all too easily. Avoid them if at all possible!
- Cheese, guacamole and sour cream: go easy! Do I need to say more?

## PIZZA

Two of the best:
- Tuna, anchovy and olive
- Hawaiian

Seafood, lean ham (but not pepperoni) or veggie options are best for weight watchers. Having half a medium pizza can save you calories over having a small individual one to yourself. Anchovies, capers and olives add taste with few calories.

*Top tips*

- Ask for your pizza to be made without cheese or with reduced-fat mozzarella.
- The thinner the base the better.
- To get the balance right, use a plate and fill half with pizza and the other half with a big pile of undressed salad.

## FISH AND CHIPS

Two of the best:
- Mini cod and chips
- Mini cod and mushy peas

On the up side, fish and chips provides protein, vitamins and some iron – it's more the huge portion sizes that's the issue for dieters.

Go for a small portion and you'll be OK. Or if you're feeling particularly virtuous, ditch the chips for mushy peas and get in another one of your five a day.

*Top tips*

- Don't eat all the batter – the soggy section underneath the fish isn't very yummy and can be discarded.
- Get dead nosey and ask what oil your chip shop uses. Beef dripping is a saturated fat but it doesn't oxidize like vegetable oil when you heat it, so it's what I prefer if having fish and chips as an occasional treat. Hydrogenated (hardened) vegetable fat will contain trans fats, the worst type for your ticker.

# Homework

We're almost at the workout bit, but before you start moving, make sure you've done your homework for this step:

- Use your food diary to work out which foods work for your waistline and health.
- Ditch sugar and dairy and educate yourself about food and nutrition.
- Experiment with ingredients and try new ones every week.
- Recognize cravings – understand where they come from and how to avoid them.

# How to Burn Fat and Shape Up

# Introduction

I'll tell you all about the exercise I do in a minute, but in the same way that I want you to educate yourself about food, you need to do the same with exercise. The bottom line is you need to be breaking a sweat for at least half an hour five times a week.

You can do more than that if you want to; I usually work out for an hour at least five times a week. I chose what works for me, but there's more than one way to crunch a crudite. If you have a dog, you can take your mutt for a brisk walk; if you're always taking the kids to the playground, use their equipment for your workout – a few cheeky chin-ups on their monkey bars, some step work on their bench and press-ups on their slide will soon have you huffing and puffing. If you've got a bike, get on it; if you're losing weight with a mate, share the cost of a personal trainer. If the kids like riding their bikes, use their speed and run alongside them. Check out your local village hall or community centre and see what exercise classes they hold. Or if you want something that's guaranteed to work and have your waistline shrinking in weeks, there are a couple of great fitness DVDs by a blonde Bristolian sexpot you can get hold of. I had a team of experts work with me on my DVDs and they both work wonders. The feedback I've had from them has been amazing. If you've bought them already, ta very much. If you haven't, what are you waiting for?

There are plenty of ways to get the old heart rate up and the metabolism going. What matters is that you spend less time sitting on your bum and more time moving it. I do what works for me, and that's what I'm going to share with you. Give it a go – but don't be scared to mix it up with something else.

I've got a mate who had a gastric band put in last year because she swore she was too busy to work out and lose the weight the right way. She runs her own business and said she couldn't spare the time or money for gym membership or a personal trainer. We went out for dinner six months after she had the band put in and it took her four hours to eat a meal. She told me it takes her that long almost every day to eat. I'm not one to throw stones – each to their own and all that – but I couldn't help but wonder how she's managed to find up to four hours every day to sit and eat when she couldn't spare half an hour a day to get off her lovely bum and move around more. I was pretty sure the money she'd spent on the gastric band could have paid for more than 200 personal training sessions or five years' gym membership. We all have our excuses, but just how valid are they when looked at under a microscope? Chances are, not very.

# TEN

# Getting Started

I'd tried personal trainers in the past. There was one – who shall remain nameless – who called me a very rude word I can't possibly repeat (but it rhymed with 'blunt') because I wouldn't run flat out for as long as she wanted me to. I gave it all I had, my body ached, I could hardly breathe, I was tired from an hour-and-a-half session and she had the audacity to tell me I wasn't working hard enough for her. I ended up throwing my water bottle at her feet – although I wish I'd taken the lid off first – and stomping out of the park.

Before our $H_2O$ Hiroshima, the trainer had accused me of not being serious about losing weight because I wouldn't try as hard as she wanted me to. She had no idea I *was* going flat out – or as flat out as the old me could go. You see, most personal trainers have never battled with the bulge. They're all mesomorphs or ectomorphs – athletic birds or skinny Minnies who have never worried about their weight, have never had to hide their lumps and bumps, and have never struggled with motivation. That's probably why they became personal trainers – because they're physically naturally suited to it.

At the time I thought my trainer was the devil incarnate, but with hindsight, how could she ever have known the difficulty involved in making a 16-stone frame do double-time squat jumps or sprint for a minute flat out? Lugging excess weight around makes you far less mobile; she thought I was lazy and apathetic, but what she was asking was actually physically impossible for me. She was a natural athlete telling a natural porker to work beyond my capabilities. I tried my hardest and pushed my body to its limit, and there she was calling me all the names under the sun because she didn't think I was working hard enough.

When I was finally ready to try again, after my wake-up call, I decided on my exercise of choice and found a trainer – and then spent weeks procrastinating about what trainers to buy and which leggings would be best before turning up for my first session. I used any excuse I could to delay the onset of the inevitable. It's like when you know your MOT is going to cost you a fortune: you can make an excuse and cancel the appointment, but at some point you're going to have to bite the proverbial bullet, get it done and pay the money. It's the same principle when your body needs a service.

When I could finally avoid my fate for no longer, like a condemned woman I packed my gym kit and drove to meet my personal trainer James. I'd lifted nothing heavier than a kettle for years; the sight of kettle bells filled me with fear. An hour-and-a-half later I crawled back to my car, hurting, humiliated and almost in tears, wondering whether I'd just made the biggest mistake of my life. I honestly felt like I'd hopped to hell and back over hot coals and razor blades. I moved more in that first session than I had for years. I jumped, squatted, ran and crunched like a Hollywood A-lister. Doing all that at nearly 17 stone and being a smoker to boot, I honestly thought I was going to expire.

But in addition to the physical pain, I felt emotional pain too: humiliation. I was sure James was looking at me with disgust. I felt like I had to explain why my body was the way it was. Apologize for being so overweight and disgusting. Make excuses for all the extra stones I'd packed onto my frame unnecessarily. I didn't actually apologize, and of course I didn't need to. James saw it as an opportunity to help me change my life, not to judge me – though I was at such a low ebb that it took me a while to see it.

But despite bursting into tears when I gingerly lowered myself into the car and glugged from my water bottle, I also felt my very first glimmer of hope in a long time. I'd done it. I'd really done it. My first session was over and I was still breathing – albeit like I needed an iron lung. I'd taken the first step on the road to a new me. It had been bloody hard, but it hadn't killed me and I felt stronger for it.

The feeling of pride soon gave way to terror when my phone rang minutes later and James told me he wanted to see me again the same time the next morning. I thought I'd ease myself in gently and do an hour a week to start off with, but he told me he'd been testing me and pushing me hard during that first session to assess the shape I was in physically. He promised me my body could take it and I'd thank him for it in the long run. He wanted to strike while he thought my enthusiasm was hot and had planned three sessions for the first week. I fumbled around for an excuse, stuttering over my words as I tried to think of which relative I could pretend had kicked the bucket, but in the end I had no choice but to meekly agree.

I learned plenty of valuable lessons after that first session – when the fear of a heart attack subsided, that is, and I'd stopped hyperventilating.

1. The first cut is the deepest. Getting off your backside and breaking into a sweat for the very first time will always be the hardest step on the road to losing weight and getting fit. It only gets easier from here.

2. Invest in a good sports bra. I looked like I was auditioning for a *Benny Hill* sketch in those first few sessions.
3. No one in the gym or down the park gives a toss about you. They're not staring at you (unless your sports bra is rubbish); they're more likely to be wondering why you're staring at them.
4. Be proud. Don't let feelings of shame override the fact that you're trying. Remember: this is about the future, not the past.
5. Turns out kettle bells are way heavier than kettles and don't make tea.

# Keep an Exercise Diary

In the same way you've been keeping a food diary, I want you to write down exactly what exercise you're doing, on which days, and for how long. You should keep a note of your fitness level in each session – how many reps you can manage in the gym, how far you can walk or jog, how many laps you can swim. Set yourself targets to reach and don't worry about how little you can do at the start – stick with it and you will do better. Keeping the diary will help you stay motivated, and you'll feel brilliant when you see what you've achieved and how you've improved over the weeks. As soon as something becomes easy, set new targets and push yourself further.

If you find yourself getting bored, look back at your diary and see if you've become stuck in a rut exercise-wise and need to try something new.

Write down how you feel after each session – it could be that your workout goes better at certain times of the day.

# No-Exercise Exercise

Even when I don't get to the park, on my bike or down the pool, I still burn fat. How? Through NEAT, or Non-Exercise Activity Thermogenesis. It's the exercise we do that isn't actually exercise in the formal sense of going to the gym or getting hot and sweaty, and it's very important in determining whether we're overweight or not. NEAT is all the time we spend shuffling and shifting in our seats, standing up, walking around, getting the kids' juice, going upstairs, downstairs and back up again because you forgot what you needed and so on. And here's the very interesting thing: it's yet another area that might be related to our genes.

A study at the Mayo Clinic in Minnesota examined weight gain in sixteen non-obese adults who were purposely overfed by roughly the equivalent of two Big Macs a day for eight weeks, while keeping their level of structured exercise (like the gym) constant. Unsurprisingly, all of these subjects gained weight. But there was a huge variation in individual response to this overfeeding: some individuals gained as little as 1.4kg, while others gained as much as 7.2kg. What the scientists found is that NEAT was the factor that accounted for much of the variation in fat gain. In other words, when overfed, some individuals naturally burned more calories through moving about more and even just fidgeting, and this increase appears to be completely subconscious and genetic.

Another study undertaken at the same clinic determined that if obese individuals had NEAT levels similar to the 'lean' subjects in the overfeeding experiment, they would burn an additional 350 calories a day – equivalent to roughly 1lb of fat every 10 days!

The take-home message from all this? Some of us are just

more predisposed to high levels of NEAT than others. But now you are aware of the possibility that you might just be less of a fidget than your skinny-Minnie friend, you can make a conscious effort to move more on a daily basis. In other words, it's not just sweating it out down the park for an hour that's important, but also all the other stuff – even small things like walking about while you're on your mobile, getting off the bus a stop early or walking to the next stop before you get on it, taking the stairs rather than the lift, sitting up straighter and getting up for a few minutes every hour you spend sitting at your desk. It all adds up and can make a significant difference in the long term.

# ELEVEN

# High-Intensity Exercise

Over the years I've tried all manner of exercise regimes, workouts and fitness classes, from Pilates to pole dancing; but after *those* pictures appeared, I opted for HIIT (High Intensity Interval Training) combined with slow resistance training. I'm not one for hours spent on the exercise bike or power walks in the park – though if you are, be my guest. HIIT works on the principle that the exercises that make up your workout should be brief, infrequent but intense.

So, if you're going to run, sprint hard for thirty seconds, then jog slowly for a minute while you recover. If you're going to squat, go hard and fast until you think you're going to wet your knickers, then walk for a minute until you get your breath back. If you're doing push-ups, go hard for thirty seconds until you think your arms are going to give out on you, then cycle for a minute until you recover and your heart stops pounding in your ears. If you're skipping with a rope, make like Muhammad Ali and go so fast the rope becomes a blur, then skip like you're in a playground for a minute to let your legs recover. The fundamental point of HIIT is to bring your heart rate up as high as it can go for a short burst before bringing it back down again.

When I was rested up in bed with my broken ankle, I watched a *Horizon* documentary called 'The Truth About Exercise'. It really opened my eyes about how our bodies work mechanically and the most effective forms of exercise for health, fitness and muscle definition.

I grew up watching Mr Motivator while eating Mini Babybels and Discos. I thought exercising meant slogging it out for ages in a gym and being one of those weird gym freaks with a six-pack, sweating buckets while evangelically telling the world you had to work hard and long to get fit. HIIT works on none of those principles. You do short blasts of working out and bring your heart rate up as high as you can, then you bring it back down for a little rest and do the same thing all over again.

The cycle of intense exercise then recovery takes your body into fat-burning overdrive mode, which enables you to carry on burning fat for up to two days after exercise. Two days! I'm always one for a quick fix, and the thought that the fat-burning party isn't over once you step off the treadmill totally appealed to me. It's so quick: you can do a workout in twenty minutes that can last you two days. It seemed a perfect fit for my anti-slogging-it-out-in-a-gym stance. HIIT sheds fat twice as fast as your average gym session – what's not to love?

Slogging it out for hours in the gym can cause your muscles to break down if you're not careful, especially if you do endurance sports, and the longer the exercise period the more prone you are to injuries over a prolonged period of time. I watched the long distance runners at the Olympics and I just wanted to cook them a good, hearty meal. HIIT training, on the other hand, can help increase speed, power and endurance, and also boosts your natural resting metabolic rate, which will help you burn fat faster and lose weight even when you're not working out. I use HIIT all the time, along with cycling, the occasional jog and some yoga. If I know I've got a photo shoot coming up, I'll use it more frequently, as it tones me up far faster than anything else. I've introduced it to tons of my mates and all their biggest fat-loss transformations have come from HIIT.

But don't take my word for it. Try it for yourself with the workouts below. Do the first workout two or three times in the first week, then switch to the second workout and do that two or three times a week for a fortnight.

### Workout 1

Spend 3 to 5 minutes warming up: start with a fast walk, then speed up into a low-intensity light jog, gradually increasing your speed.

Do one minute of moderate or high-intensity exercise: sit-ups, press-ups, skipping, sprinting or cycling. Then do one minute of low-intensity exercise such as a light jog. Repeat this routine 6 to 8 times. Don't push yourself too hard or get to the point where you're likely to cause an injury.

Spend 3 to 5 minutes cooling down: start with a fast walk, then speed up into a low-intensity light jog, then gradually decrease your speed. That's a 26-minute workout which will help you continue to burn fat for at least 24 hours.

### Workout 2

1. 3–5 minutes warm-up and stretch
2. 30 seconds sprinting, 1 minute jogging
3. 45 seconds sit-ups, 1 minute jogging
4. 60 seconds press-ups, 1 minute jogging
5. 90 seconds sprinting, 1 minute walking
6. 60 seconds sit-ups, 1 minute jogging
7. 45 seconds press-ups, 1 minute jogging

8. 30 seconds sprinting, 1 minute jogging
9. 3–5 minutes cool down

To me, working out now is all about increasing my metabolic rate so I can build more muscle. I don't want the bodybuilder look, but I want toned definition and to look strong, fit and healthy. Besides, the more muscle you have, the higher your metabolic rate and the quicker you burn fat.

While I have to go to the gym sometimes, I much prefer working out in the park. I loathe gym machines. Elliptical trainers and rowing machines make me want to reach for the bread bin. Don't use the fact that you can't afford a gym membership as an excuse not to do anything. I work out in the park, the playing fields or my back garden most days, and I've found you get a much nicer shape using your own body weight as a resistance tool, rather than using a gym machine. Once you're familiar with the exercises, you can start creating your own mini circuits.

Which brings me to the other part of my workout: slow resistance training. Here, if I do a press-up, I do it long and slow, taking between five and seven seconds to go down and back up again. It's tough to start off with, but slow resistance training will give you a sculpted shape and build muscle mass. It also helps with balance and core strength and makes everyday life so much easier. You'll find you can carry shopping bags more easily, you have better posture and can stand for much longer without getting backache. Lifting dumb bells slowly or doing a sit-up in slow motion will give the core of your body an incredible strength and help you avoid all manner of twists, sprains and related injuries which can be caused by having a weak middle.

When you're using a machine at the gym, you're often only working one body part, but if you're using body-weight exercises, you're working your whole body at once. Give both HIIT and slow resistance training a go and you'll be amazed at how quickly your body becomes strong, healthy and lithe.

When you start to get to know your body, you'll learn, like I did, that it's a very clever bit of kit. After having abused it for so long, I feel truly blessed that it's still in working order, let alone looking good. Over time, I've changed my relationship with food, my relationship with alcohol and my relationship with exercise, and finally I've changed my relationship with myself. For years I hated my body: I had always been fighting against it or abusing it, I didn't care what I put into it and treated it like crap. But now it's my best friend, not a mortal enemy, and when you feel like that you don't want to poison it with junk and crap and leave it slumped on the sofa watching TV all day. When it comes to your bod, you're the designer, the creator and the master. Your body can only ever be what you make it.

# Homework

You're almost there: you've tackled your eating and now you're working out. But before you go on to learn how to sustain your new life plan, make sure you've done the following:

- Keep an exercise diary: it'll keep you motivated when you see how much you improve, week on week.
- Get your first workout over with. You'll dread it, but I promise you'll feel euphoric afterwards.
- Increase your NEAT levels wherever you can.
- Buy my DVD and start shaking your bum!

# STEP 4

# A Lifetime Plan

# TWELVE

# Keeping Your Nerve and Coping with Plateaus

Your fat mates will understand what you're doing and your thin mates will try and empathize (bless 'em, though they'll never know what it's like carrying that much extra timber around). But here's the kicker: as soon as you start to shed a few pounds, your friends, be they fat or thin, will fall into two very separate camps, regardless of how much they weigh or their dress size.

Some will try to tempt you off the wagon. They'll hit you where it hurts: the one part of yourself you've always prided yourself on, regardless of your waist size – your personality. They'll do it with a laugh and a smile, but they'll tell you that the 'old' you was more fun. That the 'new' you is boring. The 'old' you would have stayed out longer, had one last cocktail or another pint, come out for a meal, ordered dessert, shared the kebab, cooked the fry-up. They may even say you've gone too far, and being 'too' slim doesn't suit you.

The other group will become your pep squad: your personal cheerleaders, who'll big you up and keep reminding you what a difference you're making to your body and your life. They'll also adopt a healthy eating regime to encourage you, and they'll be the ones who'll lend you their clothes and even give you that piece in their wardrobe you've had your eye on for ages but never thought you'd fit into. I remember when I got to my target trying on my mate Mia's clothes. She's always been a hottie and I was secretly envious of her because she could wear whatever she wanted. The day I fit into her skinnies was like winning the lottery.

When the negative comments happened to me, I started to wonder whether I was going to be like Samson and his strength coming from his long hair. What if my personality had been wrapped up in my weight all these years? What if I was losing my wit with every pound? Figuring out how much of your personality is wrapped up in the way you look is a tough nut to crack. There's no hard or fast rule; the answer will be different for everyone. In my case, my personality and my weight were inextricably linked. I'd developed a good sense of humour and great comic timing because I sure as hell couldn't get by on my looks.

In those early days, I honestly went through a few weeks when I was scared I'd become a completely different person inside if I was thin on the outside. That didn't happen, of course, but when you start out on this journey your self-esteem is so fragile you're almost looking for an excuse to ditch the whole thing and take a trip to Greggs. Everyone I know who's lost weight reaches a stage at some point when they wonder whether their detractors are right – whether it's true that you're going to be boring if you're thin.

You're not, by the way. You're going to be exactly the same person, only a few stone lighter, a shedload happier and a whole lot healthier. Your confidence will grow; your mood will be sunnier because you'll be sleeping better; you'll have more energy because you're eating better. Not to get into the finer details about how my bedroom action has changed since I lost weight, but I promise you, the difference is a revelation. You'll have more energy for one thing. When your tum and your bum start shrinking, you'll want to show them off to your bloke and when you're working out and are lighter, straddling him won't seem like a punishment. In short, you'll be liberated and if, like me, you've been big most of your life, you may well awaken a randy mare who's been hiding behind your weight all these years.

So ignore the haters, hold your nerve, keep the faith and believe you can do it. Just make sure you don't start getting all up yourself and think you're the next supermodel because you're on the way to becoming hot.

When I finally got down to my dream weight of 10 stone (which I hadn't been since I was about thirteen), I cried, laughed, cried, laughed hysterically and did cartwheels in the park until I was dizzy.

But despite all the celebrations, I didn't feel like I could exhale. It felt like my mission was only half completed. After all, I'd proved in the past I could lose weight – maybe not this much, but some. Keeping it off, however, was another matter altogether, and something I'd never managed before. Why would it be any different this time?

I've never been followed by so many paparazzi as in the months after I lost weight. They were desperate to get a shot of me at McDonald's or shoving a kebab in my face after a night out. There were plenty of people waiting for me to trip up and start gaining weight again. People waiting to say 'I told you so' and commiserate that I had gone back to my old bad habits. Even my mum wasn't sure I could keep the weight off. I had friends commenting on every morsel I ate and tutting knowingly if I ever skived off a workout, reminding me I was at the top of what could be a very slippery slope. I felt as if everyone was waiting for me to fail and end up back where I started.

You see, that's the problem with losing weight: you've spent months climbing a mountain and have finally reached the top, and just looking over your shoulder reminds you how far you've come but also how far you have to fall. There'll be a lot of people around you who think it's a temporary measure, not a total life change. They'll see it as being a fad, something you tried for a while before going back to the 'old' you – a bit like having a perm in the 1990s. They don't mean any harm by it – well, most of them don't – but we're never sure how to take people who completely change their lives. It all seems a bit too . . . successful for us to stomach.

After all, there are so many of us who want our lives to be different, so many people who want to change something, get a better job or move to a new country or retrain to do something else, but there are very few who actually get off their arse (whatever size it is) and try to change and *make* things happen, rather than waiting for things to happen to them. There are two types of people in this world: the 'cans' and the 'cannots'. I spent far too many years of my life being a 'cannot'. Now I'm a 'can'. I can stay slim; I can stay sexy; I can get the jobs I want; I can make a fitness DVD; I can launch a fitness website. Hell, I can do anything if I put my mind to it – even write a book.

## Coping with Compliments

Funnily enough, you won't be the only one who likes staring at your newly-emerging curves. People will start to notice you differently, and while your body is shedding pounds week by week, your mind will take a lot longer to catch up. You'll physically see the difference in your clothes and when you're in the buff, and you'll be able to read the difference in the number on the scales between your feet and on the tape measure around your gut and hips. But in your mind you'll stay fat for a good while after you've reached your target weight.

The closest analogy I can give you is going to bed as one person and waking up a completely different one. You'll look in the mirror and see you've physically changed, but in your head, you're still the 'old' you. You can see your waist is emerging, but that won't stop you crossing your arms over it when you sit down to try to hide it. These kinds of habits are as hard to break as any dietary ones.

You'll know you're losing weight, but you'll still decline invites to anything that sounds too strenuous or where there's the potential for people to see how big your bum is. It's a habit. You've done it for years and it'll take some time to shift. I remember walking through my local shopping centre, around a month or so before I hit my target weight, when I caught myself staring at a blonde girl I was sure I knew. I stopped and squinted (don't worry: I've got glasses since then) and it took me a split second to realize it was me. You see, you're so used to your reflection being something to avoid that it feels more than a little strange to finally see yourself looking good. Your brain will be on average about six months behind your body in your journey, so give it time to catch up.

I was inundated with compliments when I started to lose weight. Everywhere, from Twitter and Facebook to the supermarket, people would tell me I looked amazing and should keep up the hard work. I'd smile, laugh, blush and thank them for their support; but honestly, while I had a new body emerging from the layers of fat I'd hidden it under forever, in my mind I was still a size 20.

Compliments are such an encouragement to begin with. You start to feel so positive when people notice you're losing weight or looking healthier. But then they come so thick and fast you can run out of answers. Don't get me wrong: I was grateful for every kind word sent my way, in person and on the internet, especially after the vitriol I'd been used to receiving; but it takes some getting used to. I'd been complimented all my life on how funny I was – that I could deliver a punchline to a packed pub with just the right comic timing to get everyone laughing – but I'd never been told I was sexy, and for months after I lost the weight, all those words did was make me chuckle and blush with embarrassment at the attention.

When someone tells you you're looking hot, saying something like 'I know – can you believe it?!' makes you sound either big-headed or daft or a combination of the two. I wasn't used to receiving compliments and it took me months to feel comfortable accepting them. Lukey would tell me I was looking fantastic, but I'd just give him a thwack and call him a cheeky bugger or turn it into a joke about hanky-panky. I still don't feel comfortable when I'm told I look sexy or amazing. It's weird: I longed for compliments for such a long time, and then when they started to come I was completely unprepared to take them.

You see, when you're big, your self-esteem is so on the floor that you don't think you'll ever have someone, let alone a sexy bloke, look you in the eyes and tell you you're hot. So when it happens, your instinct is to deny it or bat away the attention because you're not used to it, you're not comfortable with it, you don't know how to deal with it and being praised for your looks feels weird. And because your brain is still stuck in the 'fat old you' mentality, it's even harder to deal with. I spent ages asking people if they were joking when they complimented me on my legs or bum or the fact I looked so healthy and fit.

The first time I went to a party in London when I was a size 10, I didn't know what to do with all the attention. It was completely overwhelming. I was chatted up and photographed way more than the old me would have been. I looked and acted like a right goof when a tall dark stranger started using pick-up lines on me. I was laughing away with him like a mate until my friend pulled me aside and told me the guy had spent the last hour-and-a-half trying to pull me. I'd been so sure he would go off with the skinny Minnie in the corner that it didn't occur to me I *was* the skinny Minnie in the corner!

I thought these kinds of blokes were completely out of my league because my confidence levels were still low. Despite having lost weight, I still had the insecurities of a big girl. Little by little, though, I started to get used to it, even to enjoy it. I used to long for attention from these kind of men and now it was actually happening. I'm not a cheater so I didn't go there, but realizing that my self-esteem was in a place where I wouldn't ever let myself be treated like crap by a bloke ever again was quite a moment.

Your brain will catch up eventually, just like mine did. I had a stand-up row with a woman in Morrisons recently who kept telling me I looked just like Josie, that girl that had won *Big Brother*. I told her it was me and she wouldn't have a bar of it. We went back and forth until eventually I showed her my driver's licence; but I think she still went away believing I was a fraud, some other slinky version of the big mare that had won the show.

If you have trouble accepting compliments, and immediately start putting yourself down, then think of it as being congratulated on your hard work. If someone at work praised you for a presentation you'd done, you'd take the praise at face value. This is the same thing – an acknowledgement of all the hours spent getting off your bum and down the gym.

# What To Do When You Reach a Plateau

You may know what you should be eating and how much you should be moving, but inevitably there comes a time in every weight-loss journey when the scales stop moving. Despite your almost religious devotion to working out and eating right, the number between your feet refuses to budge. Welcome to the plateau. Otherwise known as the Time You Get Dead Frustrated and Usually Fall Off the Wagon.

One of the biggest myths about big people is that we have a slow metabolism. In fact, when you're bigger, your metabolism can work faster than that of someone who's a size 8. You burn more energy in total each day just by lugging yourself around. But when you start losing weight, your metabolism slows down to accommodate your weight-loss. That's all a plateau is – your metabolism readjusting itself. There are two options when you get to a plateau: increase the rate at which you burn energy or fall off the wagon. No prizes for guessing which one is the correct answer.

The more weight you have to lose, the more plateaus you're likely to hit, as your metabolism will need to readjust itself a few times over. I hit four plateaus during my weight-loss journey. Think of plateaus as being like little devils who are sent to try your nerve, to test your devotion and determination. Don't give them the satisfaction of falling off the wagon. And whatever you do, don't start eating less – that'll slow down your metabolism even more and make the plateau last for longer, as your body will try to conserve its fat stores and hang onto whatever you put into it. As alien a concept as it seems at first, trust me on this: eating less when you reach a plateau will only keep you there for longer.

The best way to deal with a period when the scales won't budge –

no matter how many clothes you take off or how much you breathe in – is to increase your exercise regime. It doesn't have to be drastic; you're already working hard, after all. Just stay 15 minutes longer at every other workout, or finish your cardio with a 3-minute sprint before the warm down. Add a gentle 15-minute workout of fast walking or cycling on your non-workout days. See what else you can do to increase the energy you burn through NEAT (see page 223).

You need to keep your food intake level, as what you're eating is giving you the energy you need to make it through your workouts. Eating less and increasing your exercise is only going to leave you feeling faint and frustrated – it could see you keel over and knock yourself out on a kettle bell at the gym.

In addition to switching up your workout, you can change your diet – just make sure you're not eating less. Invent some new breakfasts based on the meal plans and ingredients listed earlier, or restrict yourself from buying your usual ingredients at the supermarket as a bit of a *Ready Steady Cook* challenge. You could try adding a bit more protein to your diet to curb hunger and increase your metabolism a bit.

You need to distract yourself from the temptation to give the whole thing up and go back to the old you. Changing something about your regular routine will do that. Do some research into superfoods (see page 110) and see if any of them float your boat. It was during a plateau of mine I that I discovered linseeds – they're cheap and dead tasty. I grind them up or blitz them in a blender and sprinkle them on porridge or add them to salads; there's nothing these lovely little seeds don't taste good with. They relieve PMT, help tackle heart disease, reduce your risk of cancer, arthritis and asthma, and they're packed with omega-3 fatty acids which are really important for a healthy heart, balanced mood and for the burning of body fat.

The main thing to remember is don't get dejected when the inevitable plateau happens, use it as motivation to dig even deeper and try even harder.

## THIRTEEN

# Enjoy the Journey and Celebrate Success

There were plenty of things that I found difficult on my way to Slimsville, but one of the hardest was learning to enjoy my new bod without worrying it was going to disappear or that it was a sign I was ill.

Sometimes I'd wake up in a cold sweat, convinced all the hard work I'd put into reducing my size had just been a dream – I'd gingerly touch my tum, sure I was going to find rolls of fat where my abs had been.

Or being the hypochondriac I am, I'd spend days worrying that the hipbones newly emerging from under all the layers of fat were a sure sign I was ill – seriously ill. I'd been big pretty much all my life and the only people I knew who'd managed to lose a huge amount of weight were the ones who were diagnosed with some god-awful disease. I spent ages feeling convinced I'd got cancer, like my Aunty Marie had had when I was a teenager. She'd lost a huge amount of weight just before her diagnosis and I was petrified the same thing had happened to me. I'd Google the symptoms of cancer, telling myself it was just my luck that I was getting sick just as I started to change my life.

I'd book a doctor's appointment and sit in the surgery on the verge of tears, begging him for a battery of blood tests to tell me I was well. It took me months to realize that I wasn't ill and that my transformation was down to all the hard work I'd put in. I'd learned how to cook to properly feed my body and help make it more injury proof than it'd ever been. I'd got out of bed enough mornings and gone to the park, the gym or the pool to make a real difference to the size of my waistline and the shape of my backside.

Once my doctor reassured me I wasn't dying, that I was just getting healthier and fitter thanks to my own hard work and determination, I started to enjoy the journey even more than before. I loved measuring myself and weighing myself once I got going: it's incredibly rewarding to see the weight and the inches dropping off you and the numbers in your notebook falling. But I was at least two-and-a-half stone into my weight-loss programme before I let myself go shopping.

You see, when you've been big all your life and you're suddenly getting slim, it's easy to think it's a temporary measure. That the body that's emerging isn't the 'real' you, and the 'real' you – the one that you've hated for God knows how many years – will come back sooner or later. You don't want to get too attached to your newly emerging waist in case it disappears again, much less spend money clothing it. What's the point in going to the shops if the new clothes you buy are only going to get a few wears before you're back into your tents and the things you can't fit into stay sitting in the back of the wardrobe, reminding you how close you came to being slim?

I used to hate shopping with a passion. When my best mate in the whole world, Candice, turned eighteen, she invited me and the girls on a shopping trip to Bristol. The plan was we'd all save our wages and then buy a fancy new outfit before changing into it for a night out clubbing. I spent five hours traipsing around town before coming home with . . . a hat. A hat! It was a nice hat and everything, but I don't remember the last time a beanie was de rigueur in the nightspots of Bristol. While Candice and everyone else had acquired mini skirts, boob tubes, slinky dresses, killer heels and cute clutches, I had a headpiece. OK, I saved myself a wedge of cash, but I'd have given anything to follow them into the changing rooms with an armful of clothes, trying them all on and looking at myself from all angles before deciding what I looked best in.

I'd spent forever lying to myself about what size I was. I'd refuse to pick up a size 20 and instead squeeze myself into the size 16 with the elasticated waist. Admitting you're a size 20 when you're in your teens or early twenties is about as likely as admitting you can finish four packs of Jaffa Cakes in one sitting. Most of the time I'd refuse point blank to go shopping with mates, pretending I had something else to do, but when it came to Candice's eighteenth I'd had no choice. While all my mates ended up getting chatted up that night, I found myself throwing shapes on the dance floor in my jeans and trainers.

I remember another Candice shopping trip – she's very persuasive – when I came home with a pair of shoes. As anyone who's been over a size 16 will tell you, shoes, bags, hats and scarves aren't fattist. They don't care whether you're a size 6 or a 16. Whenever I was made to go shopping, you could guarantee I'd come home with some kind of accessory rather than something substantial to wear.

I detested shopping so much I'd wear the clothes I owned until they were literally falling off me. Such was my dread of going near a changing room. I can still feel the misery and stress that arose when one particular pair of jeans finally gave up, ripping after years of wear. The thought that I'd be forced to go and buy a new pair was the worst feeling in the world. I'd spend hours walking round, delaying the inevitable task of having to pick something up and try it on. Just the thought of entering a clothes shop used to bring me close to tears. The shop assistants would be standing and staring at me like we both knew I had no place being in there – no place shopping in the same way as everyone else when I was so big. I felt more upset about ripping an item in my limited wardrobe than I did about crashing my car.

I can remember the zip on another pair of jeans breaking when I was a teenager. I hated the thought of replacing them so much that I just nicked my mum's boyfriend's jeans. But even they were tight and barely did up unless I was lying down.

When I finally started shrinking, two-and-a-half stone along the line, I forced myself into some retail therapy. The belts I owned were at their tightest notch and I looked like a member of Kris Kross with my jeans hanging off my arse. I remember trying on a new pair of jeans. I grabbed a size 16, hoping I'd fit into them, but when I did them up, there was still some excess room. I barely remembered to put my clothes on before I grabbed a pencil skirt in a 14 from a nearby rail: while I literally couldn't have moved in it before, I managed to do it up. I left the shop with about £100 worth of new clothes and a huge smile on my face. I thought I was Pammy Anderson.

But when you've spent years dressing to hide yourself, it can be hard to decide what styles will suit the newly-emerging you. Every big bird is guilty of looking at how other people dress and thinking 'if only', but when you're finally in the market to be able to dress how you want, it's hard to shift your mindset. I had got down from a size 20 to a 16, but I struggled for months to stop gravitating towards big floaty elasticated things to hide my body.

The elation I felt on that shopping trip was just the spur I needed to keep going. The incentive of being able to walk into a shop and pick things up off the rail like everyone else was all I needed. I didn't take my treat day for another three weeks after that. Making sure you celebrate the journey as much as the destination will keep you on the right path. Don't wait until you're at your target weight before you shop for the new you. Of course you don't want to spend a fortune, because hopefully you'll be getting smaller still, but make sure you celebrate your changing body with the odd splurge at the shops as well as indulging yourself with the foods you love on treat days. You're measuring yourself and writing things down religiously, but the numbers will mean so much more when you manage to pour yourself into a dress you've had your eye on, or a pair of skinny jeans you'd only have dreamed about six months ago. Up until now, eating will often have been the way you celebrated good news; while you can still use food as a treat and an incentive sometimes, it's about time you found something other than food to put a smile on your face and celebrate the newly-emerging you.

## Challenge the New You

Everybody needs targets. When you started this journey, you set yourself a number on the scales or a dress size, probably both, which you put on a pedestal. You set yourself a physical target, such as being able to run for a certain number of minutes or miles, keeping up with the kids on the beach, or, like me, being able to lug your mates' kids around the park when they got knackered.

You may not have reached all of your exercise targets yet, but here's the thing: move the goalposts. Don't rest on your laurels. When you feel yourself getting close to, reaching or surpassing a milestone or target, set a new one. When I started out, I wanted to be able to cycle the four miles from my house into Bristol city centre without getting out of breath. When I could feel I was getting close to that, I moved the goalposts to cycling into town and then halfway home again before getting out of puff. Then all the way home. Then when I was close to doing that, I set myself the target of cycling into town in under fifteen minutes. Moving the goalposts and challenging yourself constantly means you'll always have targets to reach, so you'll never become complacent and think, 'Oh well, now I can do what I set out to do, I can have that mega double cheese burger and watch *Trisha* all week.'

I'm easily led, though, and when I got close to my target weight, I went a bit mad taking on new challenges. I was asked to abseil off the Clifton suspension bridge for Bristol Children's Hospice. I'd normally have run a mile (not literally), but I was inspired by the kids I met and by how well my workouts were going. I was getting stronger and fitter and thought seeing somewhere familiar from a completely different angle might be interesting. I made it down in one piece – more by luck than good judgement – and while I was still trembling for about an hour afterwards, I've never been so proud of myself. I'd done something which would have been impossible for me to even attempt six months before. The old Josie, in addition to not being able to do it physically, wouldn't have had the guts to do it mentally. I was elated and delighted seeing how far I'd come, both literally and figuratively.

Since then, I've always set myself targets and when I reach them or can feel myself getting close, I set new or different ones. Right now, my targets are to complete the 50-mile round trip along the Inca Trail to and from Machu Picchu in Peru, and after I do that maybe I'll try running a half-marathon. If you don't keep challenging the new you, the one that's emerging, you'll end up lacking motivation and there's a danger you could start stagnating. And as everyone who's ever tried to lose weight knows, when you start to stagnate, you're vulnerable to reaching for the biscuit tin or the multipack of Hula Hoops.

Try something you've always wanted to do but have never had the guts to attempt. You'll feel exhilarated you did it, and the old you – the one who was big and ate rubbish – will feel that little bit further away from the new you. Changing your attitudes will help your waistline, because the more you feel like a new person, the less likely it is that the old you will reappear.

Old Josie would never have had the guts to go for it and abseil down a 90-foot sheer drop. But the new Josie jumped at the chance.

# Wiggle Room

It only takes twenty-one days to form a habit, remember, so by now eating right and exercising should be as much a part of your routine as your morning cuppa and Facebook check. If you're not there already, you're well on your way to reaching your target weight. See: I told you that you could do it, didn't I?

One of the most important lessons I've learned in the quest to keep the weight off is to give myself some wiggle room, and not to rely on the number between my feet for my happiness and self-worth. I wanted to get down to 10 stone, but when I got there, I promised myself I'd allow a 5-pound margin of error either side of my target weight without worrying or starting to feel bad about myself. That doesn't mean I'm constantly allowed to be 10st 5lb, though. Sometimes I go down to 9st 12lb and sometimes I'm 10st

4lb. Making a particular number on the scales responsible for your happiness is far too much pressure to put on yourself and far too much responsibility to give those scales. Everyone's weight fluctuates, sometimes by as much as 5lb in a day. Did you know that when it's cloudy your body retains more water because of the low pressure in the atmosphere? And you'll weigh more if you take certain over-the-counter medicines, like ibuprofen, because they encourage water retention. So it makes no sense to give yourself such a rigorous set of rules to live by. You'll only be setting yourself up for disappointment. Remember: you own your scales, they don't own you.

Giving yourself some wiggle room also means you'll be less tempted to weigh yourself constantly: the number on the scales doesn't matter that much, so what's the point of checking it with an almost religious devotion? You need to get to a place where your happiness isn't defined by your weight. Define it by how fast you can run to keep up with the kids in the park, or by how many hours you can keep dancing on a night out. Define it by how short a hemline you can get away with, or how high a pair of heels you can walk comfortably in. Define it by how many heads you turn on a night out with the girls, or by how many shopping bags you can carry home without breaking a sweat. Or by finally having the guts to go for that promotion at work you've wanted for years. After all, those are the real reasons to lose weight: to be happier, healthier, sexier, and to be around for longer. Those things are far more important than any number between your tootsies.

The other important part of getting down to your target weight is saying goodbye to the old you. For good. And really meaning it. Ditch the old clothes – and I mean *all* of them. Give them to a charity shop, or if they're anything like my old clothes were, chuck 'em straight in the bin. But make sure you get rid of the lot. Think of them in the same way as shoes: you wouldn't keep a pair of shoes that were too big for you, because it's physically impossible to grow your feet to fit into them, so what's the point of keeping clothes you'll never fit into again? They belong to the old you, and she's never coming back.

Make sure you celebrate, too. And I mean really celebrate. You've marked every milestone and given yourself treats and perks along the way, whether it be a chocolate fountain after losing the first 14lb or a facial every week for a month when you got to your halfway point, but this moment is by far the crowning glory of your journey so far. Reaching your target weight was just a dream when you started reading this book. That moment seemed like forever away and now it's finally here. Make sure you've kept the biggest and the best treat for last.

Which brings me neatly to my final lesson. Strip down to your undercrackers and stand in front of the biggest mirror you've got. Look at yourself from every angle and find three things you like about yourself. You can take as long as you need – it took me less than a minute to name my waist, legs and arms. Stand and take it all in: see how much your appearance has changed, feel the muscle tone and strength in your body, look at your clear skin and bright eyes. Smile and have a word with yourself.[†] Tell yourself whatever you want to, but make sure you congratulate yourself and really mean it. You've done really bloody well, so take a moment to drink it all in and enjoy the new you. Now get your photo diary out and take your picture. And in this one you should have the biggest smile on your face by far.

---

† Don't worry about who's listening – this is your moment, so enjoy it, sister!

# Homework

You're well on the way now, but there are still challenges to face, mantras to remember and homework to do.

- Stick to your guns: there'll always be detractors and haters, but the best way to prove them all wrong is to keep your counsel and let your body do the talking.
- Learn to accept compliments. It's OK to explain you're not used to them, but they'll start to come thick and fast, so you may as well get accustomed to them.
- Don't panic when you reach a plateau. It's a sign that things are working and your body and metabolism are adjusting to the new you.
- Celebrate and treat yourself, but make sure you keep challenging the new you. Think of short-, medium- and long-term goals that you want to achieve in the future.

# Final Letter from Josie

Well now, muckers,

There you have it: every cough, spit and whatnot on how I lost 6 stone and kept it off. If you're not there already, you're well on your way to becoming the slinky sexy mare you should have been all your life. You've already overcome some trials and tribulations and maybe the odd plateau, and no doubt you've realized you can be more determined than you once thought. Whatever you do, though, promise your Aunty Josie you won't give up. There'll be people waiting for you to slip up; your detractors will no doubt be muttering among themselves that you'll never be able to maintain your weightloss. But if this size 10 sexpot can do it, then I swear on my sweet potatoes anyone can.

You owe it to your kids, your bloke, your friends, your family and everyone who loves you to be the best version of you that you can be. Most importantly, you owe it to yourself to keep the hard work going and the weight off.

I was a heart attack waiting to happen when *those* pictures were taken and probably only a few years away from being diagnosed with diabetes. I wasn't living my life; I was just existing. I let so much slip through my fingers all those years when I was big. I didn't have the balls to go for promotions or new opportunities. Or the confidence to chat up the sexy bastard in the bar. I was too scared to stand up for myself in a lot of situations when I should have, and that's all because I was carrying too much extra timber and felt I was an easy target.

While the fat in my body coated my arteries, the fat in my mind clogged my confidence. I'm lucky it only took me until my mid-twenties to make the change, but I still feel resentful. I wasted over twenty years of my life being fat and I'll never get that time back. What should have been some of my best years were spent hiding behind my sense of humour and filling my face with crap.

I know I'll never go back to how I used to be, but if I could have been in Evans with my eighteen-year-old self when those knee-high boots wouldn't do up, I'd have said to her what I'm saying to you: 'Somewhere in an alternative universe there's a size 10 you, and she's a proper hottie. Don't leave her there!'

Lots of love,
Your Aunty Josie xxx

# Index

acne 87
additives 72
alcohol 88–9
    weekly units 89
almond milk 85, 86, 105, 115
almonds 115, 175, 176, 179
    Banana and almond lollies 175
    Choc-'o' nuts: the amazing snack
        bar 182–3
    Face lift mango and watercress iron
        power salad 147–8
    Flourless almond butter chocolate chip
        blondies 176
    Ultimate crumble 178–9
Alzheimer's disease 111
amaranth 106
anthocyanins 111
anti-inflammatory properties 110, 113
antioxidants 110, 111, 113
apricots
    I heart pork and apricot skewers 165
    Ultimate crumble 178–9
arteries 86, 111
Asian bad ass sea bass 162–3
asparagus
    Asparagus with poached duck egg and
        fresh dill mayo 142–3

    Super smoking mackerel salad
        139–40
Atwater, Wilbur Olin 70
aubergines
    Ratatouille 188
    Skinny moussaka 151–2
autoimmune conditions 107
avocadoes 113, 177
    Avocado chocolate pudding 177
    Face lift and body repair power
        salad 133
    five ways recipes 185, 186
    Grilled avocado and peachy salad 145–6
    Prawn, avocado and bacon salad 149
    Salmon with avocado and mango
        salsa 159

bacon
    Fat burning banana and bacon
        pancakes 130–1
    Maple chicken drummers 137
    Prawn, avocado and bacon salad 149
bananas 76, 80, 114, 131
    Banana and almond lollies 175
    Fat burning banana and bacon
        pancakes 130–1
    Hot mashed banana and pecans 127

bananas (*cont.*)
    Skin conditioning coconut and banana
        cold porridge  128
bean sprouts, Face lift mango and watercress
        iron power salad  147–8
beef
    Beef steak with crunchy coleslaw and
        mustard mayo  154–5
    Beefy stuffed peppers  156–7
    Chinese five spiced beef energy
        boost  170–1
    Chocolate and iron up beef stew  167–8
    Energy and iron boosting calf's liver with
        sweet potato mash  160–1
    Fillet steak with sweet potato wedges
        and herby sauce  168–9
    five ways recipes  185, 186, 188, 189
beetroot
    Energy booster power salad  141
    Super smoking mackerel salad  139–40
beta carotene  148, 157, 165
bikini, eating in your  116
biscuits  76, 79, 106, 205
bisulphites  72
bloating  79, 85, 86, 87
blood pressure
    cortisol and  33
    high  77
    lowering  111
blood sugar  33, 80, 112, 113
blueberries  111
body types  40–2
body-weight exercises  228–9
bowel movements
    IBS  107
    regular  78, 86
    and sugar withdrawal  193, 196
BPA  102
brain
    adapting to new body shape  237, 238,
        239
    and cravings  207
    effect of sugar on  84
    and feeling full  206
    fog  79

bran  77
bread  76, 78, 79
    brown  81
    granary  69
    rye  78, 106
    white  75, 77, 107
    wholemeal  77, 106
breakfast  92, 96
    recipes  127–32
    skipping  100
breast cancer  81
Breathe easy thyme and lemon BBQ crust
        chicken cold buster  153
broccoli  86
    Chinese five spiced beef energy
        boost  170–1
    Super speedy stir fry  189
buckwheat  106
bullying  49, 52–3, 54
butternut squash
    Easy chuck-in chicken stew  143–4
    Hearty happy roasted butternut squash
        soup  138–9
    Pork and poached egg spinach and
        squash salad  135–6
    Skinny bitch red prawn and mango curry
        with wild rice  172–3

cabbage  86
    coleslaw  154–5
    Easy chuck-in chicken stew  143–4
    Face lift mango and watercress iron
        power salad  147–8
cakes  79, 205
calcium  85, 86, 111, 112, 136, 175
calf's liver, Energy and iron boosting, with
        sweet potato mash  160–1
calories  69–70, 72, 73
cancer  81, 101, 102, 243
    and superfoods  110, 111, 112, 113
carbohydrates
    eating less  76–80
    misconceptions about  68–9, 70–1
    natural  75
    refined  42, 77, 204

carbohydrates (*cont.*)
  slow-releasing 42, 80
  and weight gain 77
  whole grain 77–8
carotenoid 172
cashew nuts, Choc-'o' nuts: the amazing
    snack bar 182–3
cereals, breakfast 79
challenges 247–9, 252
champagne 89
cheese 85, 86
chest congestion 153
chewing food 206
chewing gum 201, 202
chia seeds 112
chicken
  Breathe easy thyme and lemon BBQ
      crust chicken cold buster 153
  Easy chuck-in chicken stew 143–4
  five ways recipes 185, 186, 188, 189
  Maple chicken drummers 137
  Moroccan lemon chicken thighs 157–8
Chinese chilli pork salad 146–7
Chinese five spiced beef energy boost
    170–1
Chinese food 210
chips 212–13
chocolate 81, 95, 182, 183
  Avocado chocolate pudding 177
  Choc-'o' nuts: the amazing snack
      bar 182–3
  Chocolate and iron up beef stew 167–8
  craving 198, 203
  Flourless almond butter chocolate chip
      blondies 176
  Mood-lifting BBQ fruit kebabs and
      dipping chocolate 181–2
cholesterol
  good and bad 86
  reducing 115
cinnamon 152
Clancy, Abbey 39
clothes
  ditching old 250–1
  shopping for 244–7

coconut 114–15
  Choc-'o' nuts: the amazing snack
      bar 182–3
  Mood-lifting BBQ fruit kebabs and
      dipping chocolate 181–2
  Skin conditioning coconut and banana
      cold porridge 128
  yogurt 105
cod, Lemon and fennel 166–7
coeliac disease 79
cold turkey 94, 95–6, 98, 100, 194
coleslaw 154–5
colon cancer 81, 203
colour, in food 92
comfort eating *see* emotional eaters
compliments 236–9, 252
confectionery industry 81
constipation 35, 107
cooking, experimenting with 90–1, 125
corn syrup 81
cortisol 33–4, 37
courgettes
  Mixed Mediterranean veg with extra
      virgin olive oil and sea salt 186
  Ratatouille 188
cravings 73, 93, 94, 95, 96, 116–17
  how to control 196–208
  sugar withdrawal 193–6
  takeaways 209–13
Creamy spicy quinoa porridge 129
Crispy salmon with rocket salad and tamari
    dressing 134–5

dairy produce 71, 72, 85–8
  giving up 85–8, 213
dates
  Choc-'o' nuts: the amazing snack
      bar 182–3
  Ultimate crumble 178–9
depression 49–51, 52–3, 55
despair 58–9
desserts *see* sweet treats
diabetes 9, 71, 77, 81, 112, 115, 194
*Diabetes Care* 112
diarrhoea 35, 87, 107

diet pills 68
diets
    adapting to suit 92
    balanced 29, 67, 68
    experimenting with 67–8
    faddy 72
    research into 75
    short-term effectiveness 31
    *see also* Josie Gibson diet
digestive system 33, 70, 86
dinner 92
    recipes 151–74
dressings, salad 91, 92, 125
drinks
    to avoid on diet 109
    to control cravings 200
duck eggs 142–3
DVDs, workout 217–18, 229

E numbers 72
Easy chuck-in chicken stew 143–4
eaters, kinds of 21–30, 63
eatwell plate 70–1
ectomorphs 40, 41–2, 68, 219
eggs 102
    Asparagus with poached duck egg and
        fresh dill mayo 142–3
    five ways recipes 185, 186
    Pork and poached egg spinach and
        squash salad 135–6
emotional eaters 21, 27, 31, 50, 125, 199
endomorphs 40, 41
endurance sports 226
Energy booster power salad 141
Energy and iron boosting calf's liver with
    sweet potato mash 160–1
energy levels 33, 76, 79, 93, 114, 115, 234
enzymes 72, 85, 86
evolution 37–8, 78
exercise 9, 11, 16–17, 18–19, 42, 58,
    217–29
    high-intensity 225–9
    NEAT 223–4, 241
    and plateaus 241
exercise diaries 222, 229

Face lift and body repair power salad 133
Face lift mango and watercress iron power
    salad 147–8
falling off the wagon 191–2, 208, 233, 240
fat
    becoming 11–19
    being 5–9
    conserving stores of 240
    hormonally active 77
Fat burning banana and bacon
    pancakes 130–1
fat genes 36–9
fatigue 79, 87
fats
    bad 68
    good/healthy 42, 105, 113
    low-fat foods 69
fatty acids 102, 109, 112, 132, 241
fennel, Lemon and fennel cod 166–7
fermentable oligo-, di and mono-saccharides
    and polyols *see* FODMAP food group
fibre 78, 80, 111, 113, 114, 139, 152, 159,
    175, 180
    high 70, 77, 107
Fillet steak with sweet potato wedges and
    herby sauce 168–9
fish 102
    fish and chips 212–13
    white 187, 188
    *see also* cod; mackerel; salmon; sea bass;
        trout; tuna
fitness, targets 62
five ways recipes 125, 185–9
Flourless almond butter chocolate chip
    blondies 176
FODMAP food group 107
folic acid 111, 136, 143
food
    availability of 37, 38
    cravings 198, 202–5
    experimenting with 90–2, 213
    kinds of eaters 27–30, 63
    learning about 91
    relationship with 5, 11–12, 19–20, 21,
        50, 63

food diaries 61–2, 64, 78, 79, 83, 201, 213
food industry 70–1
Forever young vanilla roasted peaches 179–
   80
fridge basics 105–6
friends 233–4
fructose, naturally occurring 82
fruit
   dried 102
   Mood-lifting BBQ fruit kebabs and
      dipping chocolate 181–2
   portions per day 102
   sugars in 83, 102
   *see also* apricots; blueberries; kiwi
      fruit; lemons; peaches; pineapples;
      strawberries
FTO gene 37–8

gastric bands 218
genes 36–9, 40
ghrelin 38
GI (glycemic index) 42, 172
glucose 77, 81
   intolerance 112
gluten 79–80
gluten-free foods 80
government, dietary advice 70–1
gradual changes 96–7, 98
grains
   avoiding processed 106–7
   on diet 106
   whole 77–9, 117
granola, Homemade nut 131–2
Grilled avocado and peachy salad
   145–6
gyms 222, 223, 226, 228

habits
   changing 97
   and cravings 200, 205
   formation of 94–5, 249
   old 237
   reverting to bad 235
hay fever 87
head hunger 207

headaches 35
health 9, 54–5
   and diet 70–2
   government nutritional advice 70–1
   and refined carbohydrates 77
   sugar and 81–2
   targets 62
healthy hoggers 29
heart disease 71, 77, 81, 102, 109, 115
heart rate 68, 218, 225, 226
heartbreak 45, 46
Hearty happy roasted butternut squash
   soup 138–9
herbs 104
HIIT (High Intensity Interval
   Training) 225–7, 229
hives 87
Homemade nut granola 131–2
homework 63–4, 213, 229, 252
*Horizon* (TV programme) 226
hormones 31, 33–4, 37–8, 39
   and cravings 198
Hot mashed banana and pecans 127
humiliation 45, 46, 48, 54, 220–1
hunger
   and cravings 197
   head 207
   rating on scale 206
   recognizing false 100, 205
   stomach 207–8
hydrogenated oils 109, 213

I heart pork and apricot skewers 165
immune system 33, 81, 107, 112
Indian food 209–10
ingredients 71–2
   experimenting with 90–2, 213
   multitasking 114–15
   storecupboard and fridge 105–6
   swapping 125
inspiration 43
insulin 77, 81
*International Journal of Eating
   Disorders* 198
iodine 104

iron 110, 111, 136, 148, 160–1, 167–8, 169,
    171, 203
irritable bowel syndrome (IBS) 107

Josie Gibson diet
    cold turkey v. gradual changes 94–8
    controlling cravings 196–213
    coping with plateaus 240–2
    fat-burning and shaping-up 217–20
    foods to eat 101–6
    meal plans 117–24
    no-go foods 106–10
    recipes 125–89
    rules 99–115
    staying motivated 191–2, 235–6
    sugar withdrawal 193–6
    weeks 1 and 2 116–24
    why it works 75–98
*Journal of Nutrition* 112
juicing 89
junk food 9, 32, 47, 63, 75
    and depression 51

kale 111
kidney function 114
kilocalories 69–70
kiwi fruit, Mood-lifting BBQ fruit kebabs
    and dipping chocolate 181–2

labelling, food 29, 69, 70, 82, 83
lactose intolerance 85, 86–7, 193
lamb
    five ways recipes 186, 187
    Lamb steak with crunchy coleslaw and
        mustard mayo 154–5
    Skinny moussaka 151–2
lectins 107, 108
legumes 103, 107–8
lemons
    Lemon and fennel cod 166–7
    Moroccan lemon chicken thighs 157–8
leptin 174
linseeds 241
liver disease 81
low energy density foods 41

low glycemic index foods 42, 172
lunch 97
    high-protein 201
    recipes 133–49
Lustig, Robert 72, 80–1
lutein 111
macadamia nuts, Ultimate crumble
    178–9
mackerel 112
    five ways recipes 187
    Super smoking mackerel salad 139–40
macular degeneration 110
Magic trout pout protein bake 163–4
magnesium 110, 112, 113, 114, 136, 175,
    198, 203
mangos
    Face lift mango and watercress iron
        power salad 147–8
    Quinoa, mango and red onion
        salsa 171–2
    Salmon with avocado and mango
        salsa 159
    Skinny bitch red prawn and mango curry
        with wild rice 172–4
Maple chicken drummers 137
marinades 91, 116
Marmite 204
Mashed chilli and garlic sweet potato with
    wilted spinach 187
mayonnaise
    dill 142
    mustard 154–5
MCT (medium chain triglycerides) 105
meal plans 117–24
meals
    eating out of habit 205
    skipping 197, 204
measurements 60–1, 63, 247
meat 101, 203
    craving 203
    *see also* beef; lamb; pork
mental attitude 5–6, 9, 58–9, 62, 100, 229,
    249
mercury levels 102
mesomorphs 40, 42, 219

metabolism
    and genetics 36
    slows down at night 30
    speeding up 68, 218, 228
    and weight loss 240
Mexican food 211–12
milk 85–8
    substitutes 85, 105
    sugars in 83
millet 106
mindless eaters 27–8
minerals 77, 104, 110
mirror
    eating in front of the 116
    looking in the 59–60, 62, 251
Mixed green salad with pesto packed
    protein 185
Mixed Mediterranean veg with extra virgin
    olive oil and sea salt 186
mood swings 93, 193
Mood-lifting BBQ fruit kebabs and dipping
    chocolate 181–2
Moroccan lemon chicken thighs 157–8
motivation 43, 45–55, 58, 63, 73, 98, 100,
    222, 248
moussaka, Skinny 151–2
muscle, building 42, 76, 228

naked
    being seen 5, 7, 8
    eating semi- 116
nasal congestion 87
*National Enquirer* 52
nausea 35, 193
NEAT 223–4, 229, 241
negative emotions 58
night-time nibblers 30
non-coeliac gluten sensitivity 79
Non-Exercise Activity Thermogenesis *see*
    NEAT
nutrition, science of 72–3
nuts 70, 104
    Homemade nut granola 131–2
    *see also* almonds; cashew nuts;
        macadamia nuts; pecans; walnuts

oats 78, 106, 112
    Skin conditioning coconut and banana
        cold porridge 128
obesity
    cost of tackling 37
    and depression 6, 50–1
    rising 15–16, 37
oils
    healthy 105
    to avoid on diet 109
olive oil 125
Oliver, Jamie 14
olives, Moroccan lemon chicken thighs
    157–8
omega-3 102, 109, 112, 132, 135, 159, 163,
    164, 174, 241
omega-6 109
osteoporosis 85

palate 91
Paltrow, Gwyneth 90
pancakes, Fat burning banana and
    bacon 130–1
Parton, John James 46
pasta 76, 79
    wholewheat 77, 106
pasteurization 72, 75, 86
PEA (phenylethylamine) 182
pea shoots, Grilled avocado and peachy
    salad 145–6
peaches
    Forever young vanilla roasted
        peaches 179–80
    Grilled avocado and peachy salad
        145–6
    Mood-lifting BBQ fruit kebabs and
        dipping chocolate 181–2
    Ultimate crumble 178–9
peanuts 108
pecans
    Hot mashed banana and pecans 127
    Ultimate crumble 178–9
pepper 125
peppers
    Beefy stuffed peppers 156–7

peppers (*cont.*)
    Mixed Mediterranean veg with extra
        virgin olive oil and sea salt  186
    Ratatouille  188
    Super speedy stir fry  189
personal trainers  54, 58, 217, 218, 219–21
personality  233, 234
pesto  185
phenylethylamine  203
photographs  60, 63, 251
pills, diet  68
pineapples, Mood-lifting BBQ fruit kebabs
    and dipping chocolate  181–2
pizza  79, 212
plateaus  240–2, 252
pork
    Chinese chilli pork salad  146–7
    five ways recipes  186, 187, 189
    I heart pork and apricot skewers  165
    Pork and poached egg spinach and
        squash salad  135–6
porridge  92
    Creamy spicy quinoa porridge  129
    Skin conditioning coconut and banana
        cold porridge  128
portion control  9
positive affirmations  62, 64
potassium  114, 175
potatoes  76, 80, 103, 212–13
poultry  101
    *see also* chicken; turkey
prawns
    five ways recipes  187, 189
    Prawn, avocado and bacon salad  149
    Skinny bitch red prawn and mango curry
        with wild rice  172–4
prebiotics  143
preservatives  101
processed foods  29, 32, 70, 75, 86, 93
    meat  101
protein  70, 75, 101–2, 241
    eating more  76, 92, 93, 95–6
    portion size  100
    snacks  200
*Public Health Nutrition*  51

pulses  107–8, 108
pumpkin seeds
    Choc-'o' nuts: the amazing snack
        bar  182–3
    Ultimate crumble  178–9

quinoa  78, 106, 113
    Creamy spicy quinoa porridge  129
    Quinoa, mango and red onion
        salsa  171–2
    Super smoking mackerel salad  139–40
    Ultimate crumble  178–9

rapeseed oil  109
Ratatouille  188
raw food  70, 75
recipes  125–89
    breakfast  127–32
    dinner  151–74
    five ways  183, 185–9
    lunch  133–49
    sweet treats  175–83
red cabbage, Face lift mango and watercress
    iron power salad  147–8
relationships  6–8, 45–6, 55, 67
respiratory disorders  87
rewards  27, 192, 247, 251, 252
rheumatoid arthritis  107
rice  76
    brown  77, 106
    milk  85
root vegetables  76, 80, 90, 103

salads
    Chinese chilli pork salad  146–7
    Crispy salmon with rocket salad and
        tamari dressing  134–5
    Energy booster power salad  141
    Face lift and body repair power
        salad  133
    Face lift mango and watercress iron
        power salad  147–8
    Grilled avocado and peachy salad  145–6
    Mixed green salad with pesto packed
        protein  185

salads (*cont.*)
    Pork and poached egg spinach and
        squash salad 135–6
    Super smoking mackerel salad 139–40
salmon
    Crispy salmon with rocket salad and
        tamari dressing 134–5
    Energy booster power salad 141
    five ways recipes 185, 186, 187
    Salmon with avocado and mango
        salsa 159
salt 109, 125, 204
samphire 104
sea bass
    Asian bad ass sea bass 162–3
    five ways recipes 187
seafood 102
    *see also* prawns
seasonal foods 101
seaweed 104
seeds 104
self-belief 62, 235
self-esteem 8, 51, 52–3, 55, 58, 234, 238
setbacks 191–2
sex 7–8, 50, 67, 234–5
shopping
    and cravings 200
    for food 12–13
    for new clothes 244–7
skin
    elasticity of 82
    spots and blemishes 86, 87
Skin conditioning coconut and banana cold
        porridge 128
Skinny bitch red prawn and mango curry
        with wild rice 172–4
Skinny moussaka 151–2
sleep patterns 86, 87, 201, 234
slow resistance training 225, 228, 229
snacks, healthy 116, 197, 199
soup, Hearty happy roasted butternut
        squash 138–9
soya bean products 108
spelt 106
spices 104, 202

spinach 110, 136
    Beefy stuffed peppers 156–7
    Chocolate and iron up beef stew
        167–8
    Energy and iron boosting calf's liver with
        sweet potato mash 160–1
    Mashed chilli and garlic sweet potato
        with wilted spinach 187
    Pork and poached egg spinach and
        squash salad 135–6
    Skinny moussaka 151–2
    Super speedy stir fry 189
sports bras 222
starch 77
steak
    craving 203
    *see also* beef
stealth eaters 287–9
stomach cramps 35, 85, 87, 193
stomach hunger 207–8
store-cupboard ingredients 105–6
    to avoid on diet 109–10
strawberries, Mood-lifting BBQ fruit kebabs
        and dipping chocolate 181–2
stress 32–5, 39, 113
strokes 77, 81, 114
sugar 80–4
    addiction to 82, 84, 193–5
    cutting out 83–4, 94, 95, 109, 213
    GDA 83
    natural 75
    substitutes 105–6, 109
    withdrawal 193–6
sulphites 72
Super smoking mackerel salad 139–40
Super speedy stir fry 189
superfoods 110–15, 241
sweet potatoes 80, 90, 103, 112–13, 117
    Energy and iron boosting calf's liver with
        sweet potato mash 160–1
    Fillet steak with sweet potato wedges
        and herby sauce 168–9
    Mashed chilli and garlic sweet potato
        with wilted spinach 187
sweet treats 175–83

sweetners 109
sweets, craving 204–5

takeaways 209–13
tamari dressing 134
targets
    exercise 222
    reaching dream weight 235
    rewards for reaching 192–3, 251, 252
    setting 62–3, 64, 192
    setting new 247–9, 252
taste buds/receptors 91, 95
tea 106, 109
texture, food 92, 202
Thai food 211
'thinspiration' 43
thyme 153
tofu 108
toxic fat 34
toxins 102
treat days 73, 82, 89, 95, 99–100, 209, 247
treats
    food-based 192
    non-food based 27, 192, 247, 251
trout, Magic trout pout protein bake 163–4
tuna, five ways recipes 186, 188
turkey, Super speedy stir fry 189
Turkish food 210–11
turmeric 158
Twitter 48, 49, 52–3

Ultimate crumble 178–9
United States, dietary guidelines 71

vegetables
    on diet 103
    experimenting with 90
    Mixed Mediterranean veg with extra
        virgin olive oil and sea salt 186
    sea 104
    Super speedy stir fry 189
vision 110

vitamin A 110, 111, 112, 137, 148, 157, 165,
    180
vitamin B 111, 131, 139, 143, 147, 159, 164
vitamin C 110, 111, 112, 114, 133, 137, 147,
    148, 155, 157, 165
vitamin D 86, 135, 143, 159
vitamin E 111, 112, 113, 159, 177
vitamin K 110, 111, 152
vitamins 77, 86, 110

wake-up calls 54, 55
walnuts
    Beefy stuffed peppers 156–7
    Grilled avocado and peachy salad 145–6
watercress 111, 133
    Face lift and body repair power
        salad 133
    Face lift mango and watercress iron
        power salad 147–8
websites, food 90
weighing yourself 60–1, 63
    5-lb margin of error 249–50
weight
    defining happiness by 250
    illness related 9
Welch, Raquel 43, 76, 92
wheat 76, 77–8
Willett, Walter 71
willpower 45
wind 87, 107
workouts 227–8, 229, 241
    DVDs 217–18, 229

yogurt 72, 82, 85, 95, 105
    Super smoking mackerel salad 139–40

zinc 174